Tony Copperfield's

Primary Care

SCREAM

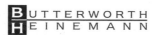

BUTTERWORTH
HEINEMANN

An imprint of Elsevier Science

EDINBURGH   LONDON   NEW YORK
OXFORD   PHILADELPHIA   ST LOUIS
SYDNEY   TORONTO
2003

Butterworth-Heinemann
An imprint of Elsevier Science Limited

For Butterworth-Heinemann:
Commissioning Editor: Heidi Allen
Development Editor: Kim Benson
Production Manager: Yolanta Motylinska

Design: Steven Gardiner Ltd, Cambridge
Printed in Spain

ISBN 0 7506 8793 2

British Library Cataloguing in Publication Data
A catalogue record for this book is available from the British Library.

Library of Congress Cataloging in Publication Data
A catalog record for this book is available from the Library of Congress.

Contents

Preface

It is easy to find a general practitioner who empathizes with the daily injustices inflicted on fellow GPs. It's relatively simple to track down a GP prepared to court controversy. It's not even that hard to unearth a GP with a flair for the written word.

But to discover someone who can do all three on a weekly basis is as rare as a social worker at 4.30 p.m. on a Friday. Except, of course, I have.

Tony Copperfield is that GP. For more than ten years he has written a regular column for *Doctor* that has inspired, enraged, challenged, entertained, understood and enlightened GPs in their thousands.

Over the years he has been reported to, and cleared by, the General Medical Council, received death threats, and generated a huge and growing postbag. Whenever he has come under attack there has always been an army of supporters ready to stand shoulder to shoulder with the great TC.

The wit and wisdom of Tony Copperfield deserves a more permanent and fitting resting place than the bottom of the nation's guinea pig hutches. Hence this collection of columns in a long-awaited book.

You asked for it, now you've got it.

Phil Johnson
Editor, *Doctor*

Each COPPERFIELD CALLING . . . actually happened and appears verbatim.

Foreword

The Americans have a saying, 'There is no Devil, there's only God when he's pissed off'

GPs are expected to play God. No-one else will volunteer and there's a distinct lack of designated funding available from central government. Besides, they're not busy.

Every week, our Satanic counterpart to the Divine cardigan wearing stereotypical family doctor takes his place at the keyboard and in 500 words or so tells it like it really is.

Health visitors who spend their entire working day in Sainsbury's coffee shop, nurses who take so much time off that their regulatory body should be known as 'Offsick', consultants who wander blindly outside their field of expertise and each and every so-called 'practitioner' who peddles bizarre quack remedies to middle-aged women gullible enough to hand over money their husbands can't afford to buy treatments that don't work for diseases that they don't have, all suffer the sharp edge of this award winning columnist's tongue.

They get off lightly compared to the knuckle-dragging halfwits who show up day after day to inflict their barrage of unsorted symptomatology and their lists of conditions downloaded from the internet onto their long suffering GP.

The release of a collection of previously published material such as this one often signals the end of a performer's creative achievement, but in Tony's case it's purely a last ditch attempt to secure a much needed pay rise from his editor. But who knows what might follow: the tour, the t-shirt, the souvenir video and special edition Volkswagen Golf?

Those of you who can still be arsed to journey from heartsink hovel to heartsink hovel to kneel in pools of vomit beside fag-burned sofas in rooms illuminated only by the light of a satellite decoder and a re-run of *Peak Practice* might find this an entertaining diversion.

The rest of you can kick off your shoes, take the battery out of your bleep and settle back with a long cool beer. The shallow end of the gene pool can be the deputising service's problem for a little while. Enjoy.

London – 1985

7.55 a.m.

Oh no. Why today? Of all the days for this to happen it had to be a Wednesday. Oh God. He had to think fast, keep calm, no point in panicking, just keep an even keel. 'The next episode will be your last.' Nothing ambiguous about that. No point being on first name terms with London's leading cardio-thoracic surgeon if you don't pay attention when he's talking to you. Oh, bollocks.

7.57 a.m.

Find the phone. Find the bloody phone. It's pitch dark in here. Find the light switch. No time, find the phone first. Under the bed, groping wildly, scattering the coffee cups, he found the dial. One finger on the stop, one finger in the zero, next finger in the nine. Shake the phone, dislodge the receiver. Oh, God this is going to be bad, really bad. Three times round, keep the finger in the hole, try not to panic. Find the cable, pull up the handset, mouthpiece covered in cold coffee. Was it his imagination or was the room really starting to spin?

7.59 a.m.

'Emergency, which service please?'
'Ambulance please, and hurry. It's 01-767-6809. 265b Blackwood Road, SW18. I've got chest pain. Horrible crushing sensations right behind the breast bone, like my chest is in a vice. Where else? It's funny, but my jaw feels numb. Really. Hurry please, it's getting worse by the minute. 265b. Thank you.'

8.02 a.m.

Find the light switch. Wait for the ambulance to arrive, can't be more than ten minutes. For God's sake get a move on.

8.18 a.m.

The traffic was already building up for the morning rush hour. Queues of commuters in shiny new Ford Sierras listening to Grahame Dene on Capital. Sirens whooping, blue lights flashing, the ambulance driver swerved and zig-zagged through red lights, around traffic islands,

1

through tiny gaps in the sea of cars and lorries opening up ahead of him. 'It has to be St Angela's, the consultant who knows me works there, don't stop at St George's, keep going, please, just keep going.' The patient in the back was starting to get panicky, better to humour him. Another six or seven minutes on the job wouldn't matter much, besides, the tea's better at St Angela's. Hope that Irish Sister is on duty. I could go for her.

Oi mate, can't you hear the bleedin' sirens then? Go on then, get up on the kerb, go on. Got a bloke here in a life and death situation and you're concentrating on the bleedin' 'Mystery Voice' competition. Wanker.

'Two sugars love, ta. So there we were, giving it beans down the Waterloo Road, Trevor's driving like he's in the RAC Rally and the bloke in the back with me seems to be in a really bad way. Looks too young to have proper serious heart stuff, I thought, but you never know. Mid to late twenties at a guess. Rambling on about Mr Fordyce knowing him inside out, how he has to get to St Angela's, how nowhere else will do. Thought about giving him a quick whiff of the gas and air to calm him down, especially when Trevor suggested diverting to George's. Arms flailing all over the place they were, couldn't make my mind up whether it was a panic attack he was having or whether he really did know enough about heart stuff to know that pain up to the jaw's a bad sign.

Either way, he wasn't having much fun. Tried to get a GTN tablet under his tongue but he spat it out, told me he'd already had three of them before we'd arrived, and that they'd only given him a terrible headache. I thought, funny that, there's this geezer heading up the Grim Reaper's garden path towards Death's door and he's worried about bleeding headaches! Was going to yell something to Trev but he's doing 65 up the wrong side of a dual carriageway at the time so thought it better not to distract him.'

'Anyway, Trev pulls in to the bay at Angela's and suddenly, our boy's up on his feet and away like a greyhound out of trap six at Walthamstow. Not a word, just up, out of the back doors and he's on his legs and disappearing through the rubber doors into A&E. Never seen anything like it. Bare-footed, in his pyjamas and voom, he's gone. I said to Trevor, 'Trev,' I said, 'he's hopped it.' We might not make much money, but we see life, eh? So Trev brings me in here for a sit down and a cup of tea. He's in there having a tête-à-tête with Sister. I'll just settle myself down here and collect my thoughts for a minute. Any more tea in the pot love?'

8.36 a.m.

Out of the ambulance. Shortcut. Got to get to Mr Fordyce before it's too late. Black rubber doors, round window in each, leading to Casualty corridor. Signposts from there, white text, green background, Radiology, Out Patient Clinics, Friends of St Angela's, Theatres. Theatres. Theatres! Down the passageway to the right, more rubber doors, green this time, then another corridor straight on. Off with the pyjama top, must look a bit odd considering. Off with the bottoms? Probably not here, come to think of it but the pyjamas will have to go. Grey sign, white text. 'Male Changing and lockers'

8.39 a.m.

Oh God. This is going to be awful. Where's Mr Fordyce? Pyjamas off. Bollock naked in Changing Room. Green cotton pants as worn by surgical teams, size Xtra Large. Green cotton top , St. Angela's logo in black ink faded by hundreds of hot washes in the hospital laundry, size Medium. No time to get picky. Both legs down one trouser leg, shit. Legs now evenly distributed, no tie up for the pants. Pants round thighs, keep legs apart, white clogs, rubber soles, standard NHS issue, Left foot size 8, Right foot size 12. Where the hell is Mr Fordyce? White dry write board, peeling black sticky tape grid; Theatre 4, Mr Fordyce, CABG. 8 a.m.

Lunchtime

'So there we were. It was our first time in theatre and we were really really nervous. Jennifer's just got hold of the retractor thing and is pulling for all she's worth to keep the ribs apart. The rest of the firm were just craning our necks for a better look. The Registrar's started to expose the left circumflex or something when there's this incredible clatter. I mean, you just had to be there and see it. Everything stops dead, you could have heard a pin drop. There's this guy, togged out in theatre greens, but they've fallen down round his ankles, so he's tripped as he's burst into the theatre and he's lying prone, or is it supine? I always get those two mixed up don't I Jenny? Heaven knows how I passed anatomy.'

Anyway, there's this bloke, flat out on the deck, arse hanging out of these huge theatre bottoms and without missing a beat, Mr Fordyce looks up from the patient's chest and says, 'This, ladies and gentlemen, is my Senior House Officer, Dr Anthony Copperfield. Regrettably Tony will be leaving us soon to pursue a career in General Practice.'

You need a bit more practice, nurse

The Department of Health says practice nurses can stand in when we go off sick. This argument is flawed, because GPs do not take sick leave. However, I have just finished a surgery which could have been handled by any life form above the functional level of the New World monkey.

No consultation needed any knowledge beyond that required to operate an automatic sphygmomanometer or to recognise colour changes on a urine testing strip. A nurse could have coped wonderfully, recommending appropriate treatment on every occasion.

Patients prefer to see nurses not because they have great warmth – if they had they wouldn't sod off and leave their caseload every time they catch a cold – but because they still find self-limiting illnesses fascinating.

I have been called into nurses' consulting rooms to give opinions on invisible rashes, normal anatomical structures – the xiphisternum is a particular favourite – and to enter a sweepstake on the life expectancy of cold sores.

Necessary skills

A nurse who had the temerity to write to a publication read by doctors said: 'Nurses have acquired all the necessary skills and training to make them more than an adequate substitute for an absent doctor.'

All the skills except two. The first talent nurses have yet to acquire is the one which tells us within seconds whether we need to concentrate on the patient or can make better use of this time signing repeat prescriptions, composing referral letters or writing a shopping list while the droning continues in the background.

Of all the techniques I teach students, the most important – nodding and grunting, giving the impression of rapt attention while concentrating on another subject – has yet to make it onto the nursing curriculum.

The second skill nurses must learn is how to suppress the desire to cover their arses. Doctors view registration as a licence to practise medicine and take responsibility for our patients' health care. Nurses view theirs as a second virginity to be protected at all costs.

Risking registration

Last weekend, I admitted a patient to one of our residential institutions. He brought his usual tablets, including one that the local pharmacy could not supply until Monday.

Because the full name of the medication was not entirely visible on the packaging the nurses felt dispensing it would put their registrations at risk.

Nurses must learn to suppress their desire to cover their own arses

I gave the patient one capsule and offered to place the remainder of the calendar pack in a sealed envelope with a note to the effect that the contents had been seen and positively identified as kosher by Dr Copperfield. Could the nursing staff give a second dose in 12 hours? I may as well have asked for a big, wet kiss.

So, if you are thinking of going off sick, just imagine a nurse locum in your chair.

'I was given these tablets – are they painkillers? The label's a bit smudged, but you can still make out "aracetamol 500mg".'

'Oh, I couldn't say. You'd better wait until the doctor gets back.'

Gaining medical insight from my car

I love my car. It's a Nissan Primera, and I point this out in case any Japanese businessman involved with a particular multinational car company happens to be reading this column and feels inspired to give me a new one.

I would be perfectly prepared to emblazon it with 'As driven by Dr Tony Copperfield' – so long as it is metallic silver with a CD player.

Unfortunately, the other day – and Japanese businessmen really need read no further – it wouldn't start.

Not only was this the first time in four years that it had failed me, it also coincided, incredibly, with the day I was taking it to the garage to trade it in for a new model – though not as new as the plush one I might get for free.

My six-year-old son provided an instant diagnosis: 'It's sad, daddy, and doesn't want to go.' I patted the little cherub on the head and pointed him in the direction of the nearest Nintendo machine as I had some serious swearing to do.

Quick service

Ten minutes later, the AA man was echoing my son's sentiments. And yes, that is extraordinarily quick service, but I wouldn't want anyone thinking this is another gratuitous piece of product placement pitching for free AA membership (see e-mail address below).

'Oh yes,' the AA man said, 'it's amazing how often this happens.' Apparently, cars consistently break down the day they are being sold. 'You see,' he explained, 'They know.'

There is, of course, a medical equivalent to this, though the underlying mechanism has only been apparent to me since his tutorial on car psychology.

How often have you encountered a previously recalcitrant smoker who has inexplicably given up the weed, only to reappear three months later with clubbing, shortness of breath and haemoptysis?

This combination of symptoms, even during autoconsult cruise control mode, is recognisable as Bad News. Why such patients are often cruelly and ironically rewarded with serious pathology had always puzzled me. Now, the answer is obvious: they already 'know'.

Too late

They have an inkling – probably the onset of ill-defined symptoms – that something is awry, and that prompts them to give up the fags. But, of course, by then it is too late.

This is not the only medical insight provided by cars. Look how often they malfunction within a week of being serviced.

There is a medical equivalent to a car breaking down the day it's being sold

And compare that with how frequently a letter from a private health organisation gushing about the high level of normality found during a health screen has to be forwarded to the local coronary care unit because the patient has had the audacity to suffer an infarct the week after his or her well-person check.

The only difference is, one scenario makes me laugh and the other doesn't.

And if you think I am about to plug private health checks to fish for a free one, you are so wrong.

But I will say cut down on referrals by sending some patients to the AA man. And buy Nissan.

Sharp idea to silence the lambs

I've got a patient on my examination couch who might have an ectopic pregnancy cooking in her right fallopian tube. I say might because I can't hear a bleeding word she's saying. There's a shrieking toddler parked six inches away from my consulting room door, hopefully suffering from the same sort of earache that she's giving everybody else within 20 yards.

The only sound-proofed feature of our open-planned nightmare of a waiting area is the wendy house, where crying children can be incarcerated while the medical staff try to concentrate on the basic bits of the job without having to resort to sign language.

I'm not going to say anything. Last time I politely asked the parent of a child, whose decibel level approached that of a Boeing 737, to cut me some slack and choose any other seat rather than the one directly outside my room, I was asked, and I quote verbatim, whether I would be happier if they waited in the f***ing car-park. Of course I would.

Continuous bawling

It will come as no surprise to any of you to learn that there are no toys in my consulting room. Anyone warped enough to bring their malevolent, snot-encrusted rug-rats into a consultation can have the job of keeping the buggers amused while I try and listen to the history of the presenting complaint above the continuous bawling of their offspring.

Besides, what is the point of spending money on Disney characters, Teletubbies and Tweenies when access to the sharps and discarded dressings bin is free and easy.

Recent research has shown that a mere ten per cent of waiting room toys harbour pathogenic bacteria. I don't know about you, but I'm not investing hard-earned folding in anything with such a pitifully low strike rate.

While Mum is prattling on about her irregular turns and funny periods, I can amuse myself watching Junior stuffing his hand into a bin full of pus-coated scalpel blades and hypodermics, fresh from the hepatitis C screening clinic.

Mood swings

In between the bits about Mum's premenstrual syndrome, the mood swings and the complaints about how hard it is to get an appointment to see me – although self-evidently it's nowhere near difficult enough – I can chuckle as I watch elder sibling, aged five and obviously not complying with the Ritalin programme, heading for younger sister, the three-year-old with the unexplained vaginal discharge, with a used syringe in his hand and an evil glint in his eye.

I can amuse myself watching Junior stuffing his hand into a bin full of pus-coated scalpel blades

'Do you have any hopes that Gavin will fulfil his obvious ambitions to get into medical school?' I ask, leaving Mum just enough time to dive full-length across the consulting room floor, sending number one son clattering into the dressings trolley, provoking an avalanche of vaginal speculae, one of which catches little sister a blow to the occiput and provokes a howl of rage.

While all this is going on, the waiting room is emptying. Peace. Perfect peace.

Copperfield's Last Theorem revealed

Hello. I'm covering Dr Copperfield's patients while he's 'away'. And I've also stepped in to salvage his column. So I'm locum and columnist. I'm a locumist.

Being a locumist isn't easy. Dr Copperfield's patients have been perplexed dealing with a doctor who shows them concern rather than the door; and it's odd encountering patients who flinch when I offer them my hand. Obviously, it's no picnic writing his column, either. Probably the best I can do is share with you a note he left which partially explains his absence.

He entitled it 'Copperfield's Last Theorem', and I quote it here verbatim:

Let X = time taken seeing patients each day two years ago and let A = time taken performing other practice tasks (eg admin) two years ago. So $X + A = T1$ where $T1$ was the time available to undertake all practice work two years ago.

Practice tasks

Let Y = time taken seeing patients each day now and let B = time taken performing other practice tasks now. So $Y + B = T2$ where $T2$ is the time available to undertake all practice work now.

B is derived by adding A (standard admin) to N, new tasks (three-monthly clinical meetings under CHD framework, audit, PCG work, clinical governance, revalidation, developing personal learning plans, and so on). N clearly tends towards infinity. And beyond.

So $B = N + A$. Substituting this into the above, we see that $Y + N + A = T2$.

But the time available now is the same as it was two years ago (in other words, T1 = T2). So X + A = Y + N + A.

Removing A from both sides of the equation gives us X = Y + N.

But as we spend the same time seeing patients now as we did two years ago, X must equal Y. This can only hold true if N = 0. Clearly, N (see above for definition) does not equal 0; as already mentioned, it tends towards the opposite: infinity. And beyond.

A PARADOX! Therefore, one of the following must be true: (1) There is a hole in the space-time continuum; (2) Euclid, Newton et al cocked up mathematical theory; or (3) We are being conned that new tasks take no time, that we can absorb work indefinitely, and that immeasurable pressure counts for nothing.

Same conclusion

At this point, there are numerous reworkings of the theorem, many vigorous crossings-out and a variety of expletives – but always the same conclusion. Then Dr Copperfield appears side-tracked down another algebraic pathway in which he states, and again I quote: 'Let A be the arse of a politician. Let D be a stick of dynamite. Let's stick D in A, light the fuse . . .' The rest is, frankly, a thought-disordered, obscene rant.

We are being conned that we can absorb work indefinitely

I cannot comment with any authority on the implications of this note. But I do know that I must end now and see some of his patients.

And when they ask 'Where is he?' I shall reply, truthfully, 'In a place where there are no sharp objects, and no calculators.'

Practise a bit of animal magic

A medical student sat in on my surgery the other day. This made me very self-conscious – partly because I wondered if he could detect the rictus I'd developed through having to be consistently nice to patients, and partly because it's hard to teach anything about medicine using punters who've got bugger all wrong with them.

I also knew that, at the end of the session, I'd have to respond to the student's incredulous expression by admitting that, yes, I do this for a living.

The only point of interest was how unconcerned the patients were to have an outsider impinging on their 'sacred' consultation. In the end, I became bored, saying: 'We have a medical student sitting in with us today, is that OK with you?'

They were so absorbed with relating the drama of their symptoms, they were oblivious to onlookers. It struck me that, for all the effect it would have, I might as well say: 'Mrs Lard, we have a sheep sitting in with us today.' So, to relieve the monotony, I did. She didn't bat an eyelid, not even when the student obligingly baaa'd from time to time.

Wildebeest option

This was fun, so we invented a game whereby the student would contrive the scenario for me to present. Thus: 'Today, Mr Brown, we're joined by a llama,' and: 'Mrs White, today's consultation will be conducted by a herd of wildebeest.'

Again, no problem. Indeed, it occurred to us that, if patients will accept consultation by wildebeest, then the shortage of orthopaedic surgeons is over, since the average wildebeest has finer dexterity and communication skills than the average orthopod. And smells better.

The point is, patients couldn't care less who manages them so long as they get adequate time to whinge and be generally pathetic. I have just inadvertently proved this. In our practice, we have devised a 'Make an appointment with' card to give to certain patients who we need to refer on to other members of the primary care team.

On this card, we tick the relevant box to indicate that the patient should book up with the chiropodist, community psychiatric nurse and so on.

In fact, this is a 'You have bored the arse off me to such a degree, I think I shall have to hurt you very badly unless you sod off and ruin someone else's life' card, but this won't fit. Besides, it keeps the punters happy by giving them something to clutch triumphantly when they leave my surgery, particularly as they never get a prescription.

Yesterday, I encountered a patient with anxiety who, a few weeks previously, I'd referred to the CPN. Except that, in the course of our conversation, it became apparent I hadn't: I had ticked the wrong box and sent her, instead, to the chiropodist.

She'd had a marvellous time offloading all her worries without interruption and getting her toenails cut into the bargain. QED. Patients don't notice and they don't care.

Patients couldn't care less who manages them, so long as they get adequate time to whinge and be generally pathetic

Anxiety management

Try it yourself. Send someone with an ingrowing toenail for anxiety management. As for me, I'm just looking forward to ticking the 'Wildebeest' box on our new appointment card. And meeting our next student.

Nurse, that's what I call a bum rap

I've never been good at keeping my vaccinations up to date. I went into medicine to be at the blunt end of the needle, pushing, rather than at the sharp end, wincing.

My practice nurses have always had to nag me into baring the deltoid for travel jabs and the like. And after my last experience, it will be a long time before I'll volunteer to be immunised against anything ever again.

It was probably my fault for introducing the concept of evidence-based medicine to the nurses during a particularly turgid clinical meeting. They promised to go and research a few topics for themselves.

A couple of days later, I found a note in my pigeon-hole. 'Tony. Just to remind you it's six months since you had your hepatitis A vaccination. If you have a second one you'll be covered until 2010. Luv, Clare, Vanessa & Sue xxx.'

Patient protection

Well, that's what I call a result. The nurses using their skills and knowledge base in a proactive manner to protect their patient against a potentially serious condition. Then again, I didn't fancy the idea of another injection, so I dragged my feet a bit. Forty-eight hours later there was another missive in the message book.

'Tony. You hardly ever take a day off sick. We don't know how you manage to stay so healthy, with all our patients coughing over you. It would be a shame if you were to contract something avoidable (say, hepatitis A) just because you couldn't find time out of your busy working day to have a teeny-weeny pin-prick. If you like, we'll stay late tonight and sort you out. C, V & S.'

My wonderful practice staff pulling together in an atmosphere of mutual support. With a tear of pride welling up in the corner of my eye as the last patient left the building, I toddled along to the treatment room.

And what a heart-warming sight it was. Not one, not two, but all three of the practice nurses had stayed behind after a busy day at the coalface. 'Hello, Tony. We've been reviewing articles about immunisation and we've found this one in *Neurology* about minimising pain associated with injections.'

Oh, my angels!

Caring concern

Off came the shirt. I was ready. 'Er, Tony, if this is going to work, we had better go gluteal.' With that, suffused with the aura of my nurses' care and concern, I hopped face down onto the couch and slid my pants down to a reasonable level. 'Will that do?' 'Oh, yes, Tony, that will do fine.'

I hopped face down onto the couch and slid my pants down

It was then that I caught sight of a copy of my column, 'You need a bit more practice, nurse', on the treatment room notice board. The next thing I saw was a full-size cricket bat swinging toward the couch. Three mighty blows later, I was too shell-shocked to move.

'There you go, Tony, all done. Bet you didn't feel a thing.'

The paper in *Neurology* showed that, if a nurse slaps the target area briskly before giving an injection, the patient doesn't feel the needle going in. Evidence-based and everything.

Truth distortion is a wheeze

I have to confess that I rarely read the *BMJ* editorials on account of them being so long, and life being so short. But I do scan them occasionally in the hope of seeing one entitled: 'The cattle prod and the consultation: now is the time'. As yet, no joy. But an editorial a few weeks ago did catch my eye. It was headlined: 'Replacing the mercury sphygmo-manometer' and I thought, that's a good idea, how about a lava lamp instead? Unfortunately, a cursory look quickly doused my enthusiasm.

Essentially, the author was suggesting that old-fashioned sphygs should be ditched in favour of automated devices. This is madness. The conventional sphyg is one of those few weapons which allows us to play patients at their own game. It lets us make things up.

You and I know that patients do this all the time. Sick-note seekers fabricate or exaggerate symptoms.

Diabetics invent blood sugar readings. Junkies devise bizarre excuses as to why they've lost their medication – a recent favourite being 'it was crushed by a passing fire engine'.

Number generators

Asthmatics are worst of all – they make everything up. They use random number generators to produce peak flow readings. They say their inhaler technique is perfect when they might as well be using the stuff as underarm deodorant. And they tell phenomenal lies about their compliance.

Research reveals that 80 per cent of patients on prophylaxis insist they use their inhalers regularly while only about 30 per cent actually do – except, apparently, in Iceland, where compliance is fantastic, presumably because, for the average Icelander, using an inhaler passes for excitement.

And if anyone is about to write to say that all this confabulation by asthmatics is simply a reflection of them all being relatively hypoxic because they're under-treated by their GPs, I say bollocks, you're lying too.

Which is why I love my mercury sphyg. It gives me the opportunity to indulge in my own bit of truth distortion. For example, it's amazing how a BP check will consistently produce a perfect result on a Friday evening when you're running half an hour late and your patient hasn't tolerated or responded to all the other antihypertensives you've tried.

I'm not suggesting I actually fabricate the figure. But I am suggesting that, if you let the mercury column fall rather rapidly, and become distracted by a stain on the ceiling at the right moment, then you can be reasonably creative with the reading you get.

I love my mercury sphyg. It gives me the opportunity to indulge in my own bit of truth distortion

Soggy sandals

So the last gizmo on earth I want is an automated BP device which not only prevents me from using my imagination but which also reveals the result to the patient.

My trusty sphyg and my untrustworthy ears mean I can get away with giving the occasional patient the thumbs-up despite their Korotkoffs indicating a two-ton systolic. There is a certain poetic justice in this, especially if they're asthmatic.

How the GMC put the pee into PR

Just when you thought you'd jumped through every hoop possible, along come the clowns from the GMC to hold one even higher.

You see, I have here the draft outline of the GMC's proposed revalidation folder – the cut-and-paste album of one year's life as a doctor, which will indicate to my 'appraiser' whether I'm fit to practise or fit for nothing.

My copy is very crumpled and I offer no prizes for guessing why. I only retrieved it from among the crisps bags and empty tinnies when I realised it might make a column.

Let me share with you some of the highlights. Here, in section B, we need details of the proportions of my time spent on clinical and non-clinical activities. Well, it was 1% and 99% respectively, but with this new bureaucratic nightmare, guess what?

In section C, I'm required to provide information about performance. Fortunately, there are subheadings to guide me, including Good Clinical Care, Keeping Up To Date (OK so far) and Relationships With Patients. As the subheading helpfully explains, this is all about 'maintaining trust' with patients. Oh dear.

Random prescription

I could try getting some diagnoses right and glancing at my computer screen to see if my randomly selected prescription fits the patient's symptoms, I suppose. I could pretend that I care deeply about the average punter's troublesome catarrh. I could practise a beseeching look that says: 'Trust me, I'm Dr Copperfield.' But it's all bollocks, obviously, so why bother?

Also under 'Information About Performance' is 'Probity'. This is fine. I'm pathologically honest, especially about the fact I don't give a toss about medicine on account of it being such a pile of crap these days, an attitude which informs both my columns and consultations.

Next, there's the predictable heap of pious bilge about how complaints have led to changes in practice – true, though, I do chuck more patients off my list than I used to.

Slick switch

And then there's the real gem: 'Describe any compliments that you have received about your practice.' I've thought hard and, yes, I do recall one patient complimenting me on how I auscultated his heart some years ago. He was particularly taken by my slick switch from diaphragm to bell over his left sternal edge.

I'd quite enjoy this section if it wasn't such utter, offensive, patronising PC shit.

Then, in section D: 'Describe any adverse service conditions that constitute a serious impediment to your ability to deliver high-quality clinical care.' They must be taking the piss. Well, one serious impediment is, as I type, being screwed up and slung back in the bin.

I'd quite enjoy this if it wasn't such utter, offensive, patronising shit

I apologise for all the rude words I've used in this column – almost my whole month's quota in one go – but it's an indication of how I feel about this claptrap. If you share my views, the solution is simple. When it arrives, bin yours too.

What can the GMC do if we all decline its PR exercise? Strike off the entire profession?

End the advice column agony

I have given up reading the problem pages in women's magazines, especially since my mate who acts as a combined agony uncle and medical adviser to one of the better known monthlies told me he gets paid to write the letters as well as the answers.

The 'real-life' problems of Traceys from Totnes and Wendys from Worcestershire are in fact the grotesque semi-pornographic fantasies of sub-editors from Surbiton and columnists from Colchester.

Still, hats off to anyone who could even conceive of some of the regrettably fictitious problems I have wet myself laughing at over the years, let alone generate some sort of reader-friendly reply.

Life will never be quite the same now I know that Melanie from Walsall, whose drug and alcohol-fuelled debauchery had been captured on videotape by her 16-year-old cousin and was available under the counter at video stores throughout the West Midlands was, in fact, the product of the warped mind of a moonlighting counsellor from Coventry.

Ethical poser

Instead, I have turned to those 'Medical Dilemmas – A Difficult Patient' articles in the comics. I even wrote a reply to one once, an ethical poser entitled: 'How I treat an old bloke who doesn't want to go to hospital to be labelled DNR' or some such. I came over all caring and MRCGP and embarrassed myself. I sank so low that I used the word 'autonomy' without irony and even suggested involving a social worker.

That is the problem with this type of article. The authors don't want to appear to be total plonkers, so they consider every differential diagnosis under the sun.

Some of us think that way all the time. One of my assistants is famous for ordering barrages of blood tests at every opportunity. Whenever I think I've caught him out, he produces a brilliant potential differential from out of thin air. I've given up trying, after the infamous 'pseudo-gout may present as swollen knee, hence the calcium and phosphate estimations' episode.

Everyday advice

What I want to see is a series of 'What I Really Do' articles, written by everyday GPs.

'Ms Stargazer, a vegetarian urban road warrior, brings her unvaccinated children, Moon Calf and Poppy Seed, to your surgery. She asks for homeopathic treatment for their asthma and scalp ringworm. How do you respond?'

In one reply I sank so low that I used the word 'autonomy' without irony

I don't know about you, but I don't view this as an opportunity for health education. Neither do I tentatively suggest a follow-up appointment in ten days. I don't consider the possibility that by declining to prescribe homeopathic remedies I might be implying criticism of a caring but misguided mother, and I don't try to explain that conventional medical treatments are safe and effective.

What I do is push the button on my desk which lights up the sign outside my door that reads 'next patient please', and use my secret weapon to drive the crusty vegan eco-fascists out.

What is it? It's a water pistol filled with Bovril. Never fails.

Doctor-whipping has to stop

These days, whenever I open a paper, tune in the radio or switch on the TV, the inevitable anti-doctor story moves me to shred paper, flush tranny down the loo or stove in TV screen with head of nearest patient. A more constructive approach might be to write an open letter to those who use these gratuitous and ill-informed swipes at our profession to fill their column inches and news programmes. So, you media tarts out there, consider these two scenarios:

One. Next time you get diarrhoea, which frankly I hope is very soon, your GP's diagnosis is likely to be gastroenteritis. With good reason – it probably is. The operative word, though, is 'probably', which translates, in medical-speak, into living with uncertainty.

There will be other pointers to suggest that your diarrhoea is a harmless and temporary bug in the system, but we GPs know there is, say, a five per cent chance that it could be the first sign of something else – such as ulcerative colitis or cancer, or something more esoteric but equally nasty.

Two choices

We have two choices. Either we share with you the unpleasant, though very unlikely, possibilities, thus scaring even more shit out of you and stimulating demands for a 'thorough check-up at the hospital', which will prove unpleasant and probably unnecessary and push up waiting lists so that those really needing them suffer huge delays. Or we take a pragmatic line, say it's gastroenteritis, safety-net with a 'Come back if it's not settling' and protect you from all sorts of anxieties by coping, ourselves, with the slight worry that we might just be wrong.

I imagine you'd favour the latter approach. Please remember this next time you run a 'He said it was just gastroenteritis – how the useless doctor missed my bowel cancer' story.

Two. It's not in our contract to be correct 100 per cent of the time, nor is it possible. Any system run by human beings will be subject to levels of error in the same way that papers mis-spell words and TV presenters fluff lines. Besides, patients and pathologies don't always oblige as much as they could – the one by failing to comply or communicate clearly, the other by declining to follow the patterns of received medical wisdom.

So what are the implications of a story in which a diagnosis is missed by innumerable doctors? That all these professionals are incompetent? That medicine doesn't measure up? No. The conclusion is that shit happens. Blame anything you like – the vagaries of illness, fate – but don't blame us.

It's not in our contract to be correct 100 per cent of the time, nor is it possible

Doctors have long been criticised for thinking they are God. Yet when we demonstrate human failings such as error, pressured communication or simply being caught out by bad luck, we are vilified further.

Battered profession

This has got to stop. Who wants to join, or remain in, a profession that has not only been knocked off its pedestal, but which is being ritually peed over by all and sundry? And who, then, will fill your precious news agendas?

Dreams reveal my fluffy soul

I am very worried. I suffer this recurring nightmare whenever I've been on holiday and am about to return to work. I'm no expert at dream analysis, but I've got an awful feeling that it means, deep down, I care about my patients. Yes, I know – it's terrible.

I realise that recounting dreams is rather tedious, but bear with me, as this one features Gail Porter and a large bottle of aromatherapy oil. It begins with me waking in bed exactly three-quarters of an hour after I'm supposed to have started morning surgery. Cut to me in my consulting room unshaven, unbreakfasted and unbelievably stressed out.

The first patient is a child flanked by various relatives who are all of the opinion that his non-appearance at school and penchant for setting fire to domestic animals is caused by ME so, obviously, they want allergy tests. My surgery is now running two hours late and, not unreasonably, the other punters have up-ended a receptionist and are using her head to batter my door down.

Of course, this dream might just mean that I'm anally retentive about punctuality. But I'm not. For example, I make a point of being ten minutes late for all meetings. This means I'm cool enough not to be constrained by something as arbitrary as time but responsible enough not to miss anything important.

George Clooney

My fantasies, as opposed to my nightmares, are fine, dandy and on-message. On my return from holiday, I want to be told by my reception staff: 'Welcome back Dr Copperfield. You're looking fit and tanned, not unlike George Clooney. There are no patients booked in for you. Why don't you relax with a coffee and I'll fetch your copy of *Loaded*.'

Doctoring skills

In post-holiday Utopia, there is no work left to do. In your absence, all your patients have switched allegiance to another doctor. Or they've all died, which is even better because it implies that they simply couldn't survive a fortnight without your superior doctoring skills and that you will remain under-employed for some considerable time.

Imagine it: your entire list dying while you're away. Statistically, it could happen – admittedly around the same time that chimp finally does type the complete works of Shakespeare. But it's the sort of thought that keeps me going.

My fantasies, as opposed to my nightmares, are fine, dandy and on-message

But these are fantasies and so are in my control. Dreams are different. My dreams are of stress and running late. And since dreams are the windows to the subconscious, I'm terrified that this all means I really have a fluffy core to my soul. Tell me I'm not alone. Answer this simple questionnaire:

1. I have the same dream as Dr Copperfield: YES/NO.
2. I am a cardie-carrying, bearded tree-hugger: YES/NO.
3. I am a well-hard cynical bastard: YES/NO.

I'm looking for a yes-no-yes combo, if that helps. I'm so grateful for your co-operation that I'll now fill you in on Gail Porter and the oil. Except I can't, because I've just realised I'm late for a meeting.

No patience for violent patients

What the hell is wrong with GPs? How did thousands of resourceful professionals get turned into a bunch of mealy-mouthed yes men who roll over and play dead in the face of adversity?

Perhaps it's just the recent media hype about bad doctors taking its toll on our collective self-esteem, but to see the way some of you behave, you might as well don a pair of comedy cocker spaniel ears, lie down with a goofy grin and wait for your tummy to be tickled.

At the time I first became a GP, a neighbouring practice decided to solve the problem of waiting times by operating endless surgeries.

Every patient who called in was seen with a proper appointment, not as quick-and-dirty walking wounded. The patients loved it, and the doctors had nervous breakdowns.

Only a second-rate bomb disposal team could have had quicker staff turnover. As for the idea that they could ever outrun patient demand, if I could spell naivete without looking it up back then, I would have carved it on their surgery door.

Unfeasible optimism

If they had the nerve to publish the results of this journey into cloud cuckoo land they might have prevented another unfeasibly optimistic practice repeating the folly – this time up in Doncaster.

A GP in Devon recommends that when faced with a drug abuser asking for extra methadone, we should ask him to swap places in the surgery so the patient is in the doctor's chair.

Great, now not only do I have a smack-head in the consulting room, I've got a smack-head with a prescription pad.

Perhaps the correct Gestalt-based therapeutic manoeuvre in that situation would be to ask the patient to imagine changing places again, so he has the problem of getting a fistful of FP10s out of the hand of a nefarious scrote on a Friday night.

But the last straw, as it so often does, came from Radio Four's *You And Yours*.

Violent threats

A perfectly reasonable GP told his interviewer that, over the years, he had been assaulted, had a disgruntled patient turn up outside his surgery wielding an axe and had his family threatened with violence if he didn't provide an unjustifiable medical certificate.

First, he said he believed his experiences were about par for the GP course. Well, I bloody hope not, or we are even deeper in the shit than I thought.

But he went on to say, and I hope I'm quoting correctly but I was choking on a bacon and egg super deep fill sandwich from ASDA that was standing in for a decent lunch: 'Of course, no one is suggesting these people should be denied access to general practitioner services.'

Abuse me, or my staff, or my family and I won't give a toss if you suffer in the gutter

Well I am. Up front, in black and white and for the record. Access to our services is a privilege and not a right. Abuse me, or my staff, or my family, and frankly I won't give a toss if you suffer in the gutter.

And what's more, I'll tell you as much to your face. You might even need some counselling afterwards.

Cervical smears, whines and videotape

Regular readers will know that I would anticipate a politically correct, patient-friendly, quasi-educational, self-indulgent, woolly and worthless activity such as videotaped consultation analysis about as much as I would relish, say, a plate of cack.

But being forced recently into a bit of videotape gazing by a bizarre set of circumstances – a trainer's absence, a registrar's anxiety about summative assessment and a bare cupboard of excuses on my part – proved inspirational.

First, it occurred to me that there must be a market for *You've Been Framed*-type video consultation howlers. Patients falling off examination couches, toddlers getting their arms stuck in sharps bins, that sort of thing.

In retrospect, I desperately regret not having a video to hand on the famous day when a telephone call interrupted a cervical smear.

Having finished the call, I absent-mindedly told the patient that she could get dressed, which was unfortunate as she still had a speculum in situ. Her bizarre and clanging gait as she made her way back to the chair really deserved to have been caught on camera.

Patient complaints

Second, I realised that video analysis etiquette could take the pain out of patient complaints.

Pendleton's Rules, in case you don't already know, are a set of guidelines for dissecting these videos and work on the 'I'll show you mine if you show me yours' principle – you share tapes, first say something nice about each other's performance and then something nasty. Now apply this principle to the in-house complaints procedure.

Patient: 'I want to complain about you refusing to visit my mother the other day.'

Me: 'Well you can't, not until you've said something nice about me.' (Shows patient guidelines for in-house complaints.'

Patient: 'Oh, I see. Well . . . um . . . that's quite a nice tie you're wearing. Now, what about you refusing to visit?'

Me: 'No, no, no. Wait. My turn. I've got to say something positive about you first. Hmmmm . . . this could take a while . . . I know! I really like the fact you've never brought a list to the consultation. That's brilliant that is, well done.'

Patient: 'Er . . . right. So. I want to complain that you didn't visit my mother. You're not fit to practise as a doctor and you should be struck off.'

Dr C: 'Good point. Now, if I may? I believe you're a sad, fat, ranting slapper and would like to share with you the thought that, during your last consultation, when you said: "What are the chances of someone stapling my stomach?" I very much wanted to reply: "None, but if you'd said your mouth, we might be able to help." Goodbye, and so glad we could resolve this locally.'

Video analysis etiquette could take the pain out of patient complaints

Safety netting

See the attraction? As for the registrar's video, it was fab. He dealt superbly with the patient falling off the couch (good safety netting, obviously), but I marked him down for trying to share decisions with the toddler whose arm was stuck in the sharps bin ('Well, we could wait and see, or we could amputate at the elbow, or . . .').

At least I can give him some tips on how to handle the mother when she complains.

It's a nursing home knockout

Do you remember *It's A Knockout*? Stuart Hall and Eddie Waring commentated as teams from seaside resorts and market towns climbed up greasy poles carrying buckets of water.

The best thing about the games was that they were more or less impossible. Any team that got even one or two balloons through the papier mâché clown's mouth would go on to the next round.

Jeux Sans Frontières had the same slapstick quality as funny foreigners in waiters' uniforms and size 19 boots clattered into the tables on a slippery turntable and dropped their plates of spaghetti.

If Stuart Hall had been with me at the Twilight Home for the Terminally Bewildered tonight, he would have chortled himself into a coma.

Ball bearings

Just like one of those puzzles where you have to get the ball bearings into the right holes, the aim of the contest was to get one doctor, one patient, the patient's named nurse, medical record and drug chart into the same room at the same time.

As Bruce Forsyth would have said: 'Good game, good game'. Except that tonight's contestants were a team from the Agency for Nurses with Special Educational Needs.

The intellectuals, defined as those nurses who can read, write, calculate drug doses and describe their patients' symptoms with something approaching accuracy over the telephone, were all on holiday.

The management roped in replacements whose sole attraction must have been a pitifully low hourly rate of pay.

Alien concept

The concept that a visiting doctor might want to set eyes on the patient he or she was asked to treat seemed alien.

Add to that the idea that they might want to look over the medical record and acquaint themselves with the patient's drug treatment prior to prescribing anything and you might as well have been speaking Japanese.

The patient was shown to her room, where we waited while number one nurse went to get the medical record.

During the second wait, while number two nurse went to find the drug charts, the patient at the centre of events decided to go for a quick whizz.

Five minutes later she was not to be found in the loo, but in somebody else's room looking bemused and wondering who the strange clothes in the wardrobe belonged to.

She was shepherded back to her own room, which by now contained the doctor, reading her notes accompanied by the wrong nurse, when the named nurse crossed the threshold carrying the drug charts dressed as a giant penguin.

At that moment, a powerful elastic band fastened to her back snapped taut and she was hauled clean out of the room across a polished floor into a vat of custard.

A charge nurse appeared, looking uncannily like Keith Chegwin

Stuart Hall convulsed with laughter as a charge nurse, looking uncannily like Keith Chegwin but fully clothed, appeared carrying a large playing card. 'We'll play our joker on this round, Doc.'

Well, OK, I made that last bit up. Chegwin was naked.

Words for when you just can't say

My favourite words in the medical lexicon are, 'idiopathic', 'lesion' and 'non-specific'. Being able to sound impressive about uncertainty is a modern art form. These fabulous words represent the materials used to create a picture which is utterly meaningless but which patients pretend to understand.

'Idiopathic' sounds fantastically technical to the uninitiated and certainly more impressive than its actual meaning, which is: 'Buggered if I know what's causing this.'

'Non-specific' is very similar. Here's how it works. If I can figure out the specific cause of your abdominal pain, then fine, I shall reward you with a diagnosis. If I can't, then it's not because of any shortcomings on my part. It's because your history or signs simply aren't good enough and so aren't worthy of any label other than the vaguely insulting 'non-specific'. Except, maybe, 'idiopathic', which is the cause of non-specific abdominal pain which recurs, obviously.

Verbal carpet

Lesion, on the other hand, is a noun, and so must mean something. The best I can come up with is that it's a 'thingy', but a thingy pronounced with a good deal of medical authority, as in the following scenario: 'So, Mrs Lard, the cause of that buzzing in your ovary when you belch in time to the theme tune of Coronation Street? Why, I suspect it's a non-specific, idiopathic lesion. Rather like yourself, in fact.'

How fantastic it is to have a convenient and imposing verbal carpet to sweep uncertainty under. And how marvellous to be able to talk utter bollocks without patients realising.

But spouting nonsense isn't confined to doctor-patient communication. Since our A&E has started to supply us with computer-generated letters listing our patients' attendances, I have started to receive a steady supply of printed garbage. I have three separate and genuine examples:

- 'Treatment: we have given the father some head injury';
- 'Diagnosis: closed fracture left brain';
- Most bizarrely: 'Principal problem – woken up saying police put in mouth. Diagnosis: distressed.

Limited dictionaries

I'd like to claim that dysfunctional and surreal communications between medical professionals are caused entirely by the vagaries of computers and their limited dictionaries. But the truth is, they're not. For example, any letter written by a consultant about a private consultation is liable to be marred by:

Idiopathic sounds fantastically technical to the uninitiated

(a) A coating of slime exuded by the specialist during the course of meeting – 'This delightful patient' – which is odd, because she was a hatchet-faced old boot when you referred her;

(b) An over-inclusive, trendy and downright bizarre diagnosis. I have enough examples to fill an entire copy of *Doctor*, but I shall restrict myself to a recent genuine case – the child diagnosed with 'attention deficit hyperactivity disorder with oppositional defiant disorder and early features of conduct disorder'. I hope they've just told him it's non-specific.

The twilight zone of old folks' homes

You might remember that a few weeks ago I had a run-in with the more sensitive members of the nursing profession. If any of you fell for the teamwork and apple-pie bullshit that turned up on subsequent letters pages, can I direct your attention to the cover of that week's *Nursing Times* where the lead story was 'How to blow the whistle on disaster docs'.

I subsequently spent a happy hour sifting through megabytes of girlie ranting in the tonycopperfield@hotmail.com mailbox. I now have enough comedy material to keep the column going for a year or two.

So, especially for the district nurse who wrote to say she'd like to see me take another pot-shot at her colleagues with impunity, here goes.

Most of us look after a nursing home and race there after evening surgery to arrive before the night staff come on.

Uniformed zombies

We know a ward round with the uniformed zombies that make up the twilight contingent is about as much fun as a rigid colonoscopy. I now realise that working permanent night shifts is a fail-safe way of avoiding continuing medical education of any kind.

Even hard-nosed deputising doctors have given up trying to make sense of it all and just scribble 'Why am I here?' on the emergency call slip, tick the box marked 'Own GP to review' and slip into the night.

Our management guru asks us to imagine a practice where things we aspire to are happening, so we can plot a course from here to there. Usually it serves to highlight the shortcomings of our current reality.

Imagine: A fax arrives from the granny-stacker giving the names of residents to be seen and a cogent reason for each request. Reality: Separate faxes arrive from all four wards. Ten minutes later, another nurse on each ward sends another fax bearing a completely different set of names or a different reason for each consultation.

Imagine: If a patient needs to be examined, they will be ready in their room, appropriately undressed. Reality: I routinely get asked to examine old ladies' swollen ankles while they are watching Jerry Springer in the television room.

Urine infection

Imagine: Nurses dealing with routine stuff as far as their expertise allows. 'Mrs Jones has symptoms of a urine infection, an MSU went off this morning. She's not allergic to nitrofurantoin, could you issue a prescription?' Reality: Every round includes two 'Mrs Jones's urine smells funny, what should we do?' consultations.

Even deputising doctors have given up trying to make sense of it all

Imagine: Residents are not described as 'chesty' if they are short of breath, feverish or wheezing. Reality: Unwell residents whose urine doesn't smell funny are routinely labelled 'chesty'.

Imagine: Repeat prescriptions are ordered from the surgery. Reality: Fit, non-chesty residents with normal-smelling urine need hand-written repeat prescriptions because their thyroxine tablets have run out. And no, I can't be bothered to argue that the half-life of thyroxine is about 50 hours and can safely be given on alternate days. Some of us have homes to go to.

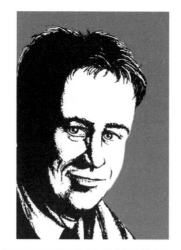

COPPERFIELD CALLING

. . . the Football Association (after England were defeated by a penalty shoot out in Euro 96)

Good afternoon, Football Association.

Hello, sorry to bother you, my name's Dr Copperfield from Essex. I wonder if I could speak to someone about my concerns for Gareth Southgate. I'm worried that he might be suffering from post traumatic stress disorder and thought that he might need some counselling. Is there someone I could speak to about this?

Hold on. (Pause). Public affairs. How can I help you?

Hello. My name's Dr Copperfield from Essex. I'm phoning because I'm interested in post traumatic stress disorder and I'm rather worried about Gareth Southgate. You know, because he missed that penalty when he really should have belted it. I wondered if anyone had offered him counselling?

Er . . . that's not really my area. Let me put you through. (Pause). Sorry to keep you. (Long pause). Hello, Claire speaking.

Hello, I'm Dr Copperfield from Essex. I'm a GP and my special interest is counselling and post traumatic stress disorder. I'm very worried about what Gareth Southgate's been going through. I'm just wondering if I could offer him some counselling?

Ummm . . . I believe he's on holiday with his girlfriend at the moment.

Is he? That's good.

So I wouldn't have thought that he'd need counselling. He's had a lot of support from his family and his friends.

So you think he's OK?

I mean, I haven't seen him since last Thursday, but he seemed fine.

Well that's good news. What about the rest of the England team? What about Gazza? We know he's a bit emotionally labile. I thought he looked close to tears again.

No, he's fine. He's just bounced back. I mean, Gareth was very upset but it's something he'll learn to live with. And, of course, Stuart Pearce has been very, very helpful.

I was very pleased for Stuart. I'm sure he's helped a lot. I bet he's terrific at counselling, Stuart Pearce.

Yes, he's the only one that really knew how Gareth felt.

So what about the supporters? Is there any help for them? You see, the BMA has just set up a help line for stressed doctors. What about all the England fans? Have there been any fans phoning up to see where they could get help and counselling?

No – we haven't had a single one phone up asking for that sort of help –

What, none at all?

No.

Well, that's something. So how do you think they should decide these matches? Penalties are just awful, aren't they?

Well, I thought penalties were pretty bad until they introduced this 'golden goal'.

Yeah . . . personally, I think they should be decided on haircuts. Eliminate those with the worst. The Czechs would never have got through then, not with Poborski in the team, would they?

Absolutely.

Anyway, it's been nice talking to you. Thanks for your help.

Bye.

Unmasking the masters of illusion

OK, I slagged off revalidation plans a few weeks ago and yes, it probably is an arse of an idea. But sometimes I revisit my opinions via moments of profound mental clarity. These are usually induced by enough Caffrey's to blot out the horrors of a surgery-load of the emotionally incontinent but not so much that I need medical attention after ill-advisedly testing myself with the Romberg manouevre (learning point for my revalidation folder: don't do this at lunch-time).

And so it was that I had a blinding insight into the reflex resistance and general brouhaha surrounding revalidation.

If we can reconcile the facts that, on the one hand, yes, we wouldn't urinate on most of our patients if they were on fire, but on the other, yes, it would be quite nice to restore public confidence if it would keep the media off our backs, then we end up scratching around for some system to achieve this.

Profound problem

Obviously, virtually all of us are pukka, but a very few let the side down. So whatever system is devised, we'll need to bow to some bureaucracy so the majority can get on with their jobs while the minority get some volts through their genitals, or whatever else the GMC decrees they deserve.

Which essentially leads us down the GMC's current path. Admittedly, the details are patronising PC bollocks, and there's the small matter of finding time, glue and pretty pictures for our revalidation scrapbooks. But I suspect there's a more profound problem at the root of our discomfort.

Revalidation will enable the public to peek into the machinations of primary care. This will reveal enormous variations in practice – not because of varying capabilities or motivations but because it is perfectly possible to function convincingly as a GP in any one of a hundred different ways. You cannot standardise primary care. Why? Because – and it hurts me to admit it – what you and I do in our surgeries every day is virtually irrelevant.

Eight-minute tricks

Such is the pointless, pitiful nature of the vast majority of problems presented to the average GP that it wouldn't matter if we managed them with antibiotics, a leaflet, a slug pellet, an impromptu rendition of the theme to *Hawaii Five-O* or the suggestion that the patient should sit on a spike for a month.

Think about your last surgery. How many patients would have come to harm had they been forced to cope without their trusted GP? In how many did your management make any real difference to what would have happened anyway?

It wouldn't matter if we managed them with antibiotics or slug pellets

The truth is 99 per cent of the time we're achieving nothing. We're treading water, we're simply finding eight-minute tricks to buy time so that nature cures or kills, or the patient loses interest before the tactical follow-up appointment.

Revalidation could lift the lid on this great illusion. I don't know about you, but I suspect this is probably not good. I've seen the future of general practice, and I need another Caffrey's.

A shot in the arm for electioneers

I know some think I'm a bit of a nihilist. My views about cervical screening and young men feeling their testicles have been aired in previous columns. One thing I do believe in, though, is the importance of giving the over-75s their annual influenza jab.

The Department of Health, which I refuse to abbreviate in any other way than 'Doh', has a massive publicity campaign to encourage everybody over the age of 65 to come forward for vaccination. A vote grabber if ever there was one.

Has anybody actually proved that immunising fit voters in their 60s makes a blind bit of difference to their morbidity and mortality rates? The 'careful review of the available data' mentioned in the circular that dropped through my letterbox sounds like a euphemism for 'fudging the figures' to me.

Hard work

The hard work, as always, will fall to primary care. Ordering the vaccine, sending out personalised letters, setting up clinics and keeping records are all considered to be the very essence of general practice. It will take no time at all.

Bollocks. GPs are currently vaccinating about half of the over-75 group each year and it's bloody hard work managing that. We are being asked to jab over 60 per cent of a much bigger target population. Where the hell are we supposed to find the time? How many routine surgeries am I supposed to cancel to make room for, let's say, a quadrupled flu vaccination workload?

Routine surgeries are one of the contractual obligations of life. It's pointless to argue that the majority of the human flotsam that turn up every day don't need to be there. Somebody has to sit through their sorry tales of life in the underclass. Until the boatload of Chinese nurses Mr Milburn has sent for turns up, we'll be kept amused doing just that.

If we can't cancel morning surgery, how can we free up the hours we would need to put into the new vaccination scheme? The clue might be in the circular after all.

Mr Milburn is offering to pay us for every vaccine we inflict on people who probably don't need it, but he won't pay us to give the vaccine to those who definitely do. Sorry Alan, but something's got to give and I bet you can guess what it's going to be.

Dubious crud

You see, it's not that we don't want to be helpful, but there simply aren't enough hours in the day, GPs at the coal face or district nurses at home on sick leave to cope with this avalanche of clinically dubious crud you're dumping on our doorstep.

Has anyone proved immunising fit voters in their 60s reduces mortality?

The last thing we want to do is to cause trouble. Honest. But if you're dumb enough to offer ready cash for an intervention with no proven benefit, we've all got families to feed or petrol tanks to fill. If there's no incentive to target the targeted properly, they'll be missed.

And the last thing Mr Blair wants to see is casualty departments full of young influenza victims in the winter before an election.

Heads would roll, Alan, heads would roll.

Getting tough on trivial complaints

You know how much I enjoy those 'How I manage . . .' bits in the medical press where GPs tell how they deal with everyday cases. I saw one the other day: 'How I manage a potential complaint', where all three of the experts wrote how they would sympathise, empathise, roll their eyes and generally bend over backwards to placate the complainant. Wrong!

Take this morning. There I was working my way through the incoming telephone calls and walking wounded when Mrs Blob storms in with all seven of her offspring in tow. Her little princess has got herself a verruca. And it's very painful. And she wants it frozen off like she used to have it done at her old doctors. And she wants it done now, not at the next cryotherapy session.

And she's not leaving until she speaks to the doctor on duty about it.

Hilarious riposte

At that precise moment, a district nurse wandered into reception. How would I feel about doing a joint touchy feely terminal care teamy assessment for one of my patients because the hospice team were on the spot and we could be there in 20 minutes?

My immediate, instinctive and frankly hilarious riposte involving a crowbar, a donkey and a tube of lubricating jelly was filed away in the mental filing cabinet for later use. I substituted an admittedly unlikely, 'Yes, I would love to'. Pausing only to ask the reception staff to tell Mrs Blob and the Blobettes that I had been called away to an urgent visit, I leapt in the car and sped off for the furthest flung outpost of our practice empire.

After half an hour or so, Mrs Blob decided not to wait to be seen. She herded her progeny home and phoned the health authority to complain about the service I offer to children in pain. They referred the call to our practice manager and she passed it to me on my return from Planet Cardigan.

According to the published experts, I should have sympathised with Mrs Blob's obvious distress, apologised for having to leave the building on urgent business, allowed her ample room to express her opinions and, by handling her complaint sensitively, should have restored her faith in my practice.

Malevolent progeny

But I didn't. I spelled things out in words of less than three syllables to ensure complete understanding at her end of the phone. I told her about our requirement that she put her complaint in writing so we could pin it up on the 'Dumb-assed Complaint of the Month' noticeboard. I informed her in no uncertain terms that the next time she dragged her litter of malevolent foul-smelling progeny into our reception area she'd better wash them first or bring a can of air freshener along to undo some of the damage.

I told her about the Dumb-assed Complaint of the Month noticeboard

And if she ever made such a fuss in the future about anything short of a near death experience she and her appalling brood would be looking for a new doctor to torment.

She was back on the phone within minutes. When was the next routine cryotherapy clinic, exactly?

When access becomes excess

Ah, excellent, a patient with a sore throat. A cursory glance, a quick fight over my refusal to prescribe antibiotics, a token threat of a complaint and, finally, my handout listing all the local GPs he might consider re-registering with.

In other words, the standard sore throat consultation, and one quick enough to get me running to time again. Except this one's different.

'I went to the chemist and he sold me some lozenges,' he begins, 'but they were useless, so I phoned NHS Direct and they advised me to see my GP. You weren't available until the next day so I saw your registrar instead. He wouldn't give me anything so I went to casualty and they took a blood test and a swab and put me on penicillin. And now I've come up in this rash.'

I contemplate this story, and his spots, for a moment. 'Why didn't you get a blue-light ambulance to take you to the nearest walk-in centre?' I ask innocently. 'Didn't you want to make a fuss?'

Blatant abuse

Five separate health professionals, two pointless treatments, two unnecessary investigations and God knows how much expense – all for a bloody sore throat.

If this chap ever gets something really wrong with him, the NHS will grind to a halt. At least he's suffering an iatrogenic rash, punishment for his blatant abuse of NHS services. There is a God of Primary Care after all.

You and I know that in Blair's Barmy New World, stories like this are becoming commonplace. They say it's all about access when in fact it's all about excess – too much healthcare, too readily available, when we could and should be toughening up the public's response to minor illness.

Instead we pander to its every symptom by providing a service with so many portals and so few barriers it borders on the obscene. By fostering a culture in which patients are encouraged not to tolerate the slightest symptom for even the briefest duration, we are creating an expensive, iatrogenic monster: the NHS itself.

Funny logic

Its going to get worse. The Man With The Plan will have us seeing all patients within 48 hours before too long. Elementary maths tells me that either we need to clone our current population of GPs, or we'll have to cut our consultation length to five minutes, encouraging open surgeries with queues around the health centre and referring everyone we can straight to casualty. Hey, that's progress.

We provide a service with so few barriers it borders on the obscene

There are, in fact, some logical alternatives. How about a system in which urgent cases are seen on the day, while patients with ongoing problems do their bit by waiting, without complaint and without coming to any harm, for the next available appointment with their trusty doc?

But stratifying urgency is difficult to convey in a headline. In a battle between logic and spin, logic always loses out. Funny, that.

'How's the throat now?' I ask, defeated, depressed.

'Still bad, he replies. 'I want to see a specialist.'

GPs' English is not the real problem here

What was that about beggars not being choosers? Here we are, ankle deep in the ka-ka with the NHS crumbling around our ears and the Tories start getting picky about the language skills of doctors in the NHS's employ. How does that square with their last great plan to solve our nursing crisis by importing ship loads from China?

Liam Fox wants 'in the interests of public safety' only to hire doctors with a sound grasp of the English language, arguing that language problems between doctors and patients may result in potentially serious medical misadventures.

Dodging regulations

He wants to try and dodge the European regulations concerning freedom of the labour market to impose a language examination on any Euro-doctor wanting to come and work in the UK. Last time I looked, there were over 20,000 doctors working in the NHS who had qualified abroad, and the vast majority of them took their medical exams in English.

Any doctor planning to work in the UK from outside the European Union has to pass both the Professional and Linguistic Assessments Board and the International English Language Testing System exam.

Dr Fox might claim that he's only trying to level the playing field so that the Dutch and the Germans have to prove their linguistic talents, but so far he's only succeeded in alienating a large proportion of the NHS workforce. Surely it can't have escaped his notice that the majority of the funny foreigners in Amsterdam and Berlin speak bloody good English.

Never mind Liam, I have a much better idea for a campaign. Why not insist that patients speak proper English during consultations, rather than taking cheap shots at our colleagues?

When you were in practice, did you get to grips with 'coming over all iffy' as a presenting symptom? When your patients complained of being 'totally monged', which chapter in the textbook did you refer to?

My assistant, who qualified in the depths of the Third World, speaks much better English than I do. His telephone opening – 'Hello, this is the doctor speaking, how might I be of service to you today?' – has the patients swooning. He also has the language problem totally sorted. Whatever the patient complains of, in whatever vernacular, they all get a standard poly-investogram of X-rays and blood tests.

When patients complained of being 'totally monged' which textbook did you refer to?

It doesn't matter whether they are banjaxed, buggered, washed out, bollocksed or shagged, they get a full blood-count, 20-odd enzyme estimations and a chest film.

Strategic migraine

The best outcome from this quasi-racist barrel-scraping crap is the suggestion that sometime next month every foreign-qualified health professional in the NHS might have a strategic migraine and spend a day watching *Teletubbies* and *Sesame Street* in an effort to improve their language skills.

We could then see how brilliantly the NHS in the inner cities would cope without them.

Verbal valium is no cure for worried well

Recognise this type of surgery? Patient one has read the information leaflet accompanying the anti-depressants I prescribed last week and wants reassuring that he will not fall foul of any of the 57 varieties of death and mayhem listed.

Patient two, aged 80, has taken note of the current vogue for testicular self-examination and is convinced he has cancer.

Patient three has just had a private screening medical and is terrified because the fawning letter from Dr Slime points out a marginally raised eosinophil count, which, despite the lack of other problems, 'you might wish to discuss with your GP'.

Patient four has hypertension, felt slightly dizzy the other day and so wants her blood pressure checked. Again.

And so on and so forth. Communal diagnosis: inappropriate anxiety.

Irrelevant leaflets

I could try telling these punters, respectively, that:

- Patient leaflets have the relevance and credibility of the average piece of junk mail and should be disposed of in the same way;
- Eighty-year-olds don't get testicular cancer and the lump is simply his normal testicle which neither he, nor anyone else, has felt for some time;
- Private screening medicals are a waste of time and money and the odd extra eosinophil is hardly a harbinger of doom;
- High blood pressure does not cause dizziness; anxiety about high blood pressure does.

But this requires a hell of a lot of effort on my part, and being a dispenser of verbal valium gets very tedious indeed.

I realise that a GP moaning about chronic neurosis is as logical and constructive as a gardener complaining that grass keeps growing. But what really pees me off is that these examples, and thousands like them, are generated by the medical profession itself – by doctors encouraging moronic preventive medicine, by the medical media supporting nonsensical campaigns and by the pharmaceutical industry writing crappy leaflets.

Stop anxiety

I have no control over the media, the private sector and the pharmaceutical industry. But perhaps primary care could take a lead in changing a culture which fosters anxiety. I'm not suggesting anything too radical – just, say, a total embargo on all preventive medicine aimed at adults.

Take blood pressure, for example. Consider the effort we put into hypertension screening, treating, monitoring, explaining, reassuring and so on. For what? Just so a handful of those we treat gain the odd extra year or two of life?

Primary care could take a lead in changing a culture which fosters anxiety

Do these patients really want a couple more years playing bingo in their dotage? And don't they waste an equivalent amount of time, in their prime, arranging doctors' appointments, BP checks, trips to the pharmacist and so on?

So save money, gain time and erase anxieties by burning your sphygs. Bring back reactive care – prevention is worse than cure.

When in Rome — specialise

I'm sorry to say that Mrs C's devotion to the art of shopping still knows no bounds. Although she has dragged the family to Italy for our holiday, at least she eased the blow by renting a villa the size of a cottage hospital. Its owner, Ronaldo, is a satirist and is very big in Italy, but then again, so are Emerson, Lake and Palmer.

On my travels I've noticed a distinct lack of two of the things that make life in Britain what it is.

First, there are no car body repair shops. It seems there is a law that no vehicle lower than a Ferrari ever gets dents knocked out of its doors. While every Testarossa is in showroom condition, every Fiat, on the other hand, has scars that demonstrate why the Italians hire a German to drive for them when it matters.

The other thing missing is general practice. Every *dottore* is a specialist. It seems to work fine, with the average Italian enjoying a long and healthy retirement, road traffic accidents permitting.

There are plenty of quacks around. My beloved is at a spa full of Americans spending money their husbands can't afford on treatments that can't work for conditions that don't exist.

The UK NHS is about 6,000 GPs short of the full picnic, and that's without making any allowance for the demographic timebomb that's going to hit us in a few years when one inner-city GP in three will hit retirement age or the 48-hour access scheme.

Favourite specialty

So, why not give up on the concept altogether?

What I am suggesting is that we doctors re-brand ourselves after our favourite speciality. It would make no real difference to our everyday work but it would really bugger the heartsinks.

If I label myself as a paediatrician – and with my uncanny resemblance to George Clooney that would be no problem – anybody wanting to see me would need to have a paediatric problem. My partners could deem themselves to be specially skilled in gynaecology, rheumatology, and so on.

I could pop off for a couple of refresher courses in child health, maybe even sit the DCH, and then devote my time to determining the exact dose of chlorpromazine elixir I would need to render that annoyingly noisy four-year-old bambino in the corner of the cafe unconscious.

But, when Mrs Scrag wants to pop in for another pointless chat about her funny turns, she'll have to track down a GP dumb enough to have designated himself as a funny turn specialist. She won't find one because none of us are that stupid.

When she wants rehousing, she'll need a housing-ologist. And that's my point. If we confine ourselves to medical matters (remember those books you spent hours poring over at medical school?), then the non-clinical stuff and nonsense will have to find somewhere else to go.

What I am suggesting is that we re-brand ourselves after our favourite specialty

Practice nurses could take on the role of 'client navigator' and within 48 hours, navigate most of the crud back onto the street where it belongs.

Non-clinical stuff

Local priests and publicans could become 'specialist counsellors' and the social work department of your friendly local authority could encroach onto the neurologists' territory by printing a batch of headed notepaper announcing its rebirth as the local teaching hospital's department of indecision and inertia.

Meanwhile, we could get on with the jobs we were actually trained to do.

Profligate pill popping pushes my patience

I regard signing repeat prescriptions as something to do with my hands while I recount to my colleagues the amusements which saw me safely through another morning of somatising cretins such as – to take my last surgery – the woman complaining of problems with her 'carnal tunnel', or the man who claimed the pharmacist had insisted he 'insult the doctor' before using OTC hydrocortisone cream.

But my grateful weeping at these solecisms is abruptly ended by the pharmacist calling to ask whether I realised I had septupled a patient's methotrexate dose by prescribing it daily rather than weekly. Oops. Maybe the suggestion to insult me was fair enough.

Tedious chore

Signing repeat scrips is such a mind-numbingly tedious chore that mistakes are bound to happen. The underlying problem seems obvious – too many patients on too many drugs.

These days a patient cannot be discharged after an infarct without a litany of statins, nitrates, aspirin, olols and oprils – and a PPI in case it was dyspepsia all along.

The pharmaceutical intake of the average diabetic is even worse. I have to hand a regime involving two different oral antidiabetics, three different anti-hypertensives, a statin and aspirin, not to mention the inhalers to help with breathlessness from carrying bags of drugs around. I know of junkies who would baulk at taking this many pills in a single day.

When I sign a prescription like this, it occurs to me that either the patient is taking, daily, 15 different tablets of seven different types at four different times of day, in which case he must be obsessive compulsive and so should be on clomipramine too. Or he isn't. I suspect the latter, on account that he's a human being and it's incredibly naive and stupid of the profession to believe anyone could cope with such a regime, particularly as none of the treatments make him feel better in any way.

How have we reached this ridiculous state of affairs? Through advances in research and the advent of EBM, demonstrating that different medications reduce morbidity blah blah blah. But we've made two fundamental mistakes in reaching these conclusions. One, that these drugs, together, have additive or multiplicative beneficial effects as opposed to, say, combining to form a nerve poison. And two, that patients are happy to absorb an endless number of pills onto their popping list. This cannot be true. There must be a limit to what patients can take, through constraints of expense, time, inclination or credulity.

But they won't tell us for fear of seeming ungrateful.

Pharmacological room

The answer is simple. Doctors should be banned from prescribing more than four drugs to any patient at any one time. If a fifth drug becomes necessary, then one of the original four has to be discontinued to make pharmacological room. Easy. And this is not a plea for the pharmaceutical industry to produce atenoaspedipinatinopril retard combinations, as these are costly and inflexible. And, besides, they'd spoil a perfectly good column.

I know of junkies who would baulk at taking this many pills in a single day

We have to be slick to survive

It's not a great time to be a doctor. According to the media, we are all either homicidal or incompetent. 'Why do heart surgeons make so many mistakes?' has replaced, 'Is your GP secretly a mass murderer?' as the tabloid theme of the season.

Confessing to cock-ups in public is suddenly fashionable and this spirit of openness means we can now entertain our friends with the harrowing stories of ghastly near misses we used to keep to ourselves.

My close encounter with the 'Deaths and Complications' meeting hinged on the meaning of the word 'reasonably'.

A medical registrar asked me to give Mr X, who cannot be named, not for legal reasons but because I've blocked out any memory of his name, an intravenous injection of verapamil 'reasonably slowly'.

Evidently, my conception of reasonable slowness didn't tie in with the patient's as his heart stopped dead about 15 seconds into the procedure. A few minutes' CPR and a couple of jump starts later, normal service was resumed and Mr X regained consciousness, asking, quite reasonably, what the hell had just happened to him.

Hapless victim

Without batting an eyelid, the registrar calmly told the hapless victim he had just had one of those nightmares that were a side-effect of the medication he'd just received. Nothing to worry about at all old chap. End of story. Mr X discharged home fit and well five days later.

So let's confess and get it over with. All doctors are psychopaths. Outwardly presentable, above average intelligence, but able to think quickly and extricate ourselves from trouble with a smile and an appropriate ad lib.

And the reason for this sociopathic majority? No other personality type has a snowball's chance in hell of making it up the career ladder.

Think back to those medical school interviews. When the panel trailed out the inevitable, 'And why did you decide to apply for a place at medical school?' question, anybody fool enough to tell the truth would have been out of the door on their proverbial pinna.

The bit about fancying four years as a student on the piss, cramming for a few months to get through finals, moving on to the serious business of driving fast cars, shagging nurses and then settling down in a five-bedroom detached house with the ward sister of my choice remained unspoken.

All doctors are psychopaths, able to extricate ourselves from trouble with an appropriate ad lib

The lying bastards who were able to spout politically acceptable bollocks about being privileged to have the ability to do their bit for the greater good were the ones that got the places. Just like me and you.

Non-stick coating

I went on to convince interview panels that I wanted to be a career obstetrician, paediatrician, geriatrician and psychiatrist to put together my training scheme. So did many of you.

So it's no surprise that when the shit hits the fan, we are good at donning the non-stick coating and making sure the reputation stays unsullied. Just call me 'Teflon Tony', physician and surgeon.

We're all in the same boat

Junior hospital doctors —don't you just love them?

Dr Copperfield: 'I'd like to send in a chap who I reckon has a leaking aortic aneurysm.'

Junior Doctor: 'What makes you think that?'

Dr C: 'Just a feeling and, oh yes, the fact that he's shocked, in agony and has a pulsatile, tender abdominal swelling.'

JD: 'What's his temperature?'

Dr C: 'Who cares?'

JD: 'Have you done a rectal?'

Dr C: 'I did one once but I didn't like it.' And so on.

I don't mind indulging in these dialogues because (a) I enjoy hearing what dumb ass questions the houseman will devise in an effort to fend off work and (b) I know I'll win. After all, if I get bored, I can use those heavily-loaded words: 'So you're saying you won't see the patient?' This is analogous to punters provoking me with: 'So you're refusing to visit?', the difference being that my ploy gets the leaky aneurysm seen while the punter's makes me dig my heels in further.

So any antipathy I feel towards junior hospital doctors doesn't stem from the Great Admissions Game, but rather to their ability to fan the flames of dissatisfaction in patients. Let's face it, the punters don't need much encouragement.

Urgent admission

For example, I was recently treating an elderly lady's chest infection with erythromycin. It soon became clear that it was time for nebulisers and nurses, so I arranged her urgent admission. To my astonishment, later that day, I received an irate phone call from her daughter.

'The doctor at the hospital said the antibiotics you prescribed were no good,' she raged. 'He said it was lucky they got to her when they did or she could have died.' Hmmm. Actually, they didn't get to her, I sent her to them, and then only after the 'Have you checked her urine?' routine and much unseemly pleading. And I was using the antibiotics recommended in the *BNF* but, hey, what's the most respected pharmaceutical reference to someone with a white coat, four weeks' experience, and Bedside Attitude? Explaining this to Splenetic Daughter is clearly a waste of time, as she's already composing her complaint, so I summarise by saying, 'Bastard'.

OK, I probably played the same game in my days as an SHO: through ignorance that GPs see illness at a confusingly early stage, through grievance at all the other crud I had to deal with, and through a desire to stroke my own ego, I would self-aggrandise at the expense of the patient's GP. I didn't realise patients and relatives would note the muttered comments, the raised eyebrows, the contemptuous sighs . . . And I didn't appreciate how they stewed on them and shaped them into venom to spit at their formerly trusted family doctor.

What's the BNF to someone with a white coat, four weeks' experience, and Bedside Attitude?

Implied criticism

So my message to junior hospital doctors is: we're all in this together. Be careful, because voiced or implied criticism is unprofessional and usually unfair – and may light a nasty fuse. Oh, and have you got an orthopaedic bed handy? I've got a houseman here with two broken legs.

An antidote for poisonous patients

Thank God for Claire Rayner. One quote from her and I am laughing no matter how bad the day has been. 'GPs and patients are now equal partners in health care.'

That's either the funniest thing I've heard in weeks or a hell of an insult to the intelligence of 30,000-odd doctors.

'Even the most poisonous patient has something to contribute,' is another one of hers, which proved eerily accurate this morning when the two-year-old from hell topped all of his previous performances by taking a dump in his pants at the start of his eight-week-old sister's well-baby check.

On an attention-seeking scale of one to ten, this scored an easy 11. Contributions don't get more poisonous than that.

I left the room to an incoming health visitor with a cheery, 'I should give that a minute if I were you' and moved on to reception.

Smiley faces

The late Mr Driver's relatives didn't like his death certificate.

I didn't know people were supposed to like them. Have I missed a memo from Claire about drawing smiley faces around the border?

How am I supposed to write an enjoyable death certificate? 'Died laughing – secondary to good sense of humour.' 'Cause of death – ecstasy'— hang on, that's one for the coroner's officer isn't it?

They didn't like 'senile dementia' as a 'significant diagnosis'. Even though the deceased was several sandwiches short of a picnic.

In my considered opinion, a single-figure score out of a possible 30 on the Mini Mental State exam ruled out any possible career switch to astro-physicist, although he may have had a future as a Patients' Association spokesman.

Demented he was and 'demented' I wrote. Except the family weren't bothered about that – it was the word 'senile' they objected to.

But dear, sweet Claire. When I'm down up she pops with a priceless 'GPs are largely to blame for their patients' failure to attend appointments'.

The scales fell from my eyes. When patients ring the surgery to book ten minutes of my time the receptionists have been getting it all wrong. 'Dr Copperfield can see you at 3.40pm on Wednesday,' they say, 'is that convenient'?

Misguided hope

Their misguided hope was that the patient would understand the question and reply 'yes' or 'no' as appropriate. I have even overheard those who have had NVQ training move on to the advanced stage by offering callers an alternative time and date if the first one doesn't suit them.

He topped all of his past performances by taking a dump in his pants

But all this time, mild-mannered patients have been meekly accepting appointments at ludicrous hours like 10.50am on Tuesday. No wonder they don't turn up.

How, exactly, should we play it? Why not call their bluff? 'Dr Copperfield will see you at 4.15am next Friday. You won't be at work, collecting the kids from school or doing the weekly freezer centre run. You'll miss *Football Italia* on Channel Four. Sometimes you just have to make sacrifices.'

If I really didn't care, you'd know it

As if the punters don't have enough weapons in their armoury already — demands, lists, the body odour of a yak and so on – they've managed to dream up another. That is, they've taken to accusing me of 'not caring'.

Quite where they've got this idea from, I can't imagine. Maybe it's just practice population gossip; maybe not, though. While 'Dr C has started prescribing antibiotics' or 'Dr C gave me a housing letter' certainly would be big news locally, 'Dr C doesn't care in the community' is more mission statement than revelation.

Alternatively, perhaps the punters have suddenly developed such powers of perception that they can successfully peek into the dingiest recesses of my psyche. But I somehow doubt that, as here we are dealing with a population who usually can't see beyond the ends of their own runny noses.

Stroppy unwashed

Whatever. A few of the stroppy unwashed seem to think that this barb will hurt where all other have failed.

Case one: a patient wants a cough mixture for her URTI-afflicted toddler on the basis that: 'Our last GP was so kind that he'd never let us leave the surgery without some medicine.' I decline.

Case two: a patient with nothing wrong but longstanding anxiety wants referral to a specialist for tests – again. I refuse.

Case three: a patient has seen an alternative therapist who has recommended tests and treatment which I think are nonsensical. I say 'no'.

Each has led to a verbal or written complaint, the crux of which is that I don't care.

Wrong. I don't cure, I don't concur and I don't collude, respectively. But if I really did not care, then I wouldn't bother to do my job properly and so I'd prescribe indiscriminately, overload the hospital with unnecessary work and not worry about causing iatrogenic harm in patients.

In fact, all these things are more important to me than how patients choose to interpret my actions. I care about needs not wants.

Accusations of not caring simply stiffen my resolve. If patients cared about their doctors, though, they'd choose their words more carefully, as other personalities might react differently.

Average cardie

For example, the average cardie might be feeling a bit moist around the eyes and wondering if the NHS occupational health scheme runs to post-traumatic stress counselling yet.

Not me. My attitude is simple. Any patient who doesn't think I care, doesn't deserve to be cared for by me.

Accusations from patients of not caring simply stiffen my resolve

They can insult me all they like, they can gossip and slander in the waiting room, they can deluge me with complaints and they can tut at my lack of vocation – even as I try to secure an urgent appointment at the hospital on their behalf, or as I remove a lost tampon before breakfast on a Sunday duty.

Yet for all this, they may report me to the GMC for my attitude and the GMC will probably take them seriously. See if I care.

If you don't laugh, you'll cry

I confess: I don't usually bother to look away from the computer screen or my copy of *Maxim* during the emergency clinic. It's so rarely worth the trouble and, besides, if the patient really is ill he or she can always come back tomorrow and see the registrar for a proper 25-minute 'fit-in' consultation.

So I don't know what it was that distracted my attention from a three-page spread of that blonde from *Brookside* in her underwear. Probably the fact that the kid on his way into my consulting room was limping like Quasimodo with a stone in his shoe.

I pay even less attention to speakers at PGEA meetings than you do, but I do remember that one of them once made it very clear that you should never ignore a limping child.

So I didn't. I did the whole thing: history, examination —looking, feeling and moving —and finally came to the conclusion that I hadn't the faintest idea what was wrong. I even checked his shoe for pebbles just in case. No history of trauma, no fever or signs of sepsis, just a knee joint that pointed 20 degrees out of true.

Clueless parents

Was his knee like this last week? No one had noticed. Older brother thought it might have been but couldn't be certain. Mum and Dad, as would become apparent later on, did not have a clue.

'Has he hurt himself last night or today?' A definite no to that one. I moved into concerned physician mode and told his parents I was going to phone a specialist for advice.

'I know what you're thinking, doctor,' said Mother. As I wasn't actually thinking of anything specific at the time I knew she had to be wrong, but I didn't imagine she'd be quite so far off course.

'He had a hamburger yesterday and now he can't walk properly. It's BSE, isn't it?'

I know you aren't supposed to piss yourself laughing at moments like this, but there are occasions when you just can't get out of the room in time. You do your best, but the glottis and nostrils can't hold it in.

Unlike those times when you're certain to throw up and it is just about possible to divert, there's no point in sniggering into a metal waste-paper bin because all that does is lend the laughter a sinister resonance.

His parents were so dim they wouldn't notice if his leg fell off completely

So I corpsed. I was still giggling when the registrar got around to answering his bleep. Which was just as well, as no amount of reasoned argument could persuade the registrar to take a peek in tomorrow's outpatient clinic.

'It sounds like synovitis.' No it didn't. 'There's probably an effusion.' No there wasn't. 'He must have had a viral infection last week.' No he hadn't. 'Give him some ibuprofen and see what happens.' You win – your wish is my command.

Limping patient

So off the patient limped, dragging his foot behind him and giving it the full Igor, with nothing approaching a diagnosis, and accompanied by parents so dim they wouldn't notice if his leg fell off completely unless they were buying shoes for him at the time.

'Next.'

Fifteen seconds and counting . . .

Fifteen minutes? Fifteen minutes! The last time I indulged in a 15-minute consultation was when I was a trainee and still believed that patients complaining of 'tired all the time' might actually have something wrong with them.

So when a colleague told me of the latest Big Appointment Idea, I assumed he'd misheard, and the real target was 15 seconds. Seeing punters at this rate would give us some hope of achieving the appointments-within-48-hours challenge.

And much can happen in 15 seconds. Local lowlife can stink out the room, psychotoddlers can wreck the place, and so on. In view of these Essex biohazards, my partners pride themselves on speed consulting. One works so fast that he can deal with a list, rattle off a scrip, check the BP, take an opportunistic smear, explore issues of previous sexual abuse and, briefly, empathise, all in roughly the time it took you to read that sentence.

Proudest moment

In fact, my proudest moment as a GP involved a very brief intervention. A new patient registered and insisted her young son had to be seen instantly as an emergency.

As it turned out, the child simply needed a repeat prescription for Wysoy for a dubious-sounding milk allergy. I pointed out that seven-year-old children don't need prescriptions for milk substitutes and her definition of the word 'emergency' needed realigning.

So she went out and deregistered. From registration to consultation to deregistration in one minute. See what can be achieved with a little effort?

But no. They really do mean 15 minutes, and this time it's not Government PR but our own GPC cranking up patient expectations. Which begs the question, what space–time continuum is the GPC working in?

In some parallel universe, maybe I'd enjoy nice long consultations so I could get to grips with the fascinating story of Mrs Lard's catarrh —although, frankly, I can think of better ways to spend 15 minutes of my life expectancy, and narrative-based medicine is unrewarding when narrated out of someone's arse.

Besides, real life dictates otherwise, unless we increase waiting times or double the number of doctors – or halve the number of patients, which will require some seriously attractive culling.

Main problem

If this system is implemented, the main problem I will have is filling those long, empty minutes between patients. Even I have a limit to the amount of Hobnobs and coffee I can consume, so I'll have to devise ways of keeping the punters talking to pad out the time. I might start saying to them, 'While you're here, patient, do you think I could check your cholesterol and feel your prostate?'

My partners pride themselves on speed consulting

I might ask them if they can find a list for me to go through or a magazine article to discuss. I might say: 'Your child sounds a bit chesty, why don't we fit him in and have a little listen, you can't be too careful?' I might even say: 'Tiredness, hmmmm. Sounds interesting. Tell me more.' On the other hand, I might just renew my subscription to *Viz*.

When action is better than words

You might think I never read the blue comics, but I'd be an idiot to ignore the pages of column-fodder that drop through my letter box every week.

The arrival of the college journal invariably sparks off a feeding frenzy as I dig into its comedy goldmine for inspiration, but now the *BMJ* has come up trumps.

As soon as I read the first sentence of 'Personal View', I knew I was in for a treat – 'I am a psychotherapist.'

There are worse people in the world, such as rapists and axe murderers, but at least they don't try to earn a living from their activities. You don't see child molesters touting for business in the personal ads or writing columns for the Sunday supplements. Besides, the criminally insane freely admit they set out to maim, corrupt and mislead, unlike psycho-babblers, who claim to help their victims despite a massive body of evidence to the contrary.

The anonymous author had a big problem, namely a sarcoma eating through the tissues of his hand. Even I felt some sympathy – sarcomas are pure evil in cellular form.

Goodbye metacarpal

Showing appropriate respect for the diagnosis, the surgeon called the patient in to his clinic ahead of time and broke the news, followed by the only information that anyone in his situation needed to hear – that it was treatable.

Goodbye metacarpal, goodbye tumour. Regrettably, goodbye little finger. Hey, you can't make an omelette . . .

Round about now I would have been running a lap of honour around the grannies queueing for a hip replacement. I would have been planning a celebration, big style.

Which is why I'd never make it as a psychotherapist, because the next item on his agenda was to analyse the consultation as though it were a chat about choosing wallpaper. Was this some sort of power game? What effect did he think he was having on me? Why didn't he ask about my work? Because in the real world, it doesn't bloody well matter.

Excellent excision

Whether you are a dustman or a concert pianist, if you make it through surgery for the mother of all malignancies and can't go back to your old job, you train for a new one. Thank God it was a pinkie and not a femur, and move on.

'It's my hand, not yours.' What kind of adolescent thought processes underscored that little outburst? 'It's my ball and I'm going home?' Is it because psycho-analysts never make anyone better, so they feel threatened when they meet someone who can? The surgeon was as good as his word, and performed an excellent excision.

Even I felt some sympathy – sarcomas are pure evil in cellular form

Only a tree-hugger wouldn't realise that asking an orthopaedic surgeon to show empathy is like asking Jeremy Clarkson to go easy on vegetarians. I'm sorry that meeting someone who knows his job and does it well was such a frightful experience.

I'd recommend a session of post-traumatic debriefing, if it hadn't been shown to do more harm than good. Why not just enjoy feeling hurt, angry and frustrated for a few decades? Or get over it.

Alternative medicine my eye

'And do you know what, doctor? Just by looking in my eyes he could tell I had arthritis in my hips and knees.' She leans back with an air of triumph and awaits my reaction. And they say this iridology stuff is nonsense!

Well, it is, because this lady is 85 years old, and divining wear and tear in her joints is about as impressive as predicting that, under the purple rinse, her hair might be grey.

Faced with this nonsense, I tend either to mock-collude with an exaggerated 'marvellous!', or simply hum and haw non-committally. Any other reaction eats seriously into the patient's sad beliefs and the consultation's seven minutes.

Occasionally, though, I just can't stop myself. The suggestion from a private osteopath to a patient of mine with chronic low back pain that she must continue to see him 'weekly for the rest of her life' was, I felt, a manipulation too far.

I have nothing against osteopaths. We employ one in our practice, but the patient gets three strikes and is then out – on the basis that if a short course of pummelling hasn't helped then there's no point continuing.

Blank cheque

As I explained to my patient, her private osteopath's management strategy appeared to involve her writing him a blank cheque – a ploy likely to help her back only in that it would lighten any strain caused by carrying money.

To be fair, most alternative practitioners seem less callous exploiters of patients' vulnerabilities than well-meaning individuals with bizarre health beliefs. If they weren't healing my patients they'd end up doing counselling or feng shui, so society is probably better off with them sticking to tweaking toes and making nice smells.

Enthusiasts will, of course, point to some evidence: the *BMJ* printed a paper 'proving' that homoeopathy is of significant benefit in treating rhinitis. The real conclusions to be drawn from this are that the *BMJ* is letting political correctness cloud editorial common sense – and research science isn't all it's cracked up to be.

The latter view stems from the philosophy of a colleague who believes that if something appears implausible, it doesn't matter what the evidence says – it's still implausible. Such is OBM (opinion-based medicine), a new school of thought with which I'm proud to be associated.

My opinion is that alternative medicine is, essentially, bollocks. References: none. Meta-analysis: lots of jumbled-up thoughts in my head. If you don't accept this, I'll use the opinion-based GP's technique of repeating myself, but louder.

Isn't it suspicious that iridologists specialise in soft illnesses with high placebo responses?

Placebo response

Besides, doesn't it strike you as suspicious that the iridologists and reflexologists specialise in soft illnesses with high placebo responses?

I'll stick to my opinionated views until I see an alternative practitioner achieve something when a patient has a real illness. I anticipate with interest the trial on foot massage versus cardiac massage for patients with cardiac arrest.

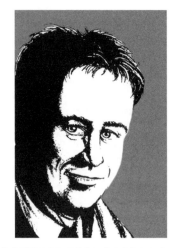

COPPERFIELD CALLING

... *a private plastic surgery clinic*

Hello, clinic.

Hello, my name's Dr Copperfield from Essex. I wanted to speak to someone for advice about one of the operations you offer.

Ah, I'm afraid you've just missed the doctors – they've gone out for a meeting. Could you call tomorrow?

Possibly . . . are there no other people who could speak to me?

Well I might be able to help.

It's about a friend of mine who's after this operation to extend the length of his penis.

Penoplasty.

Yes . . .

I could send you some details. And the cost.

Is there no information you can give over the phone?

Well, you fire away and I'll try to answer.

How is it done? And how much longer will it be?

Ah . . . it really is a little awkward. Let's send you some stuff – I'll call back tomorrow.

Hello, clinic.

My name's Dr Copperfield. I wanted to talk to somebody about – er penoplasty.

Yes, we do that here.

Is there anyone there who can help me?

Sure, no problem.

You? I ask you, do I?

Er no, not me, I'll pop you through to somebody. Is it for yourself?
Um . . . a friend.
OK, just hold the line a minute. Was it Mr or Dr Carson?
Copperfield. Dr Copperfield. Obviously Mr Carson has a problem too.
Ha ha. No. Just someone I spoke to earlier on. No excuse. Just hold the line. (Pause). It's engaged. Shall we call you back?
God no. I mean, no thanks. I'll hold. (Long pause).
Hello.
Oh hello, sorry to bother you. My name's Dr Copperfield. I'm just enquiring on behalf of a friend. A friend who wants his penis enlarged. I just wondered if you could give me some details on how it's done and cost. I imagine a bit is sort of grafted on from somewhere or something.
No . . .
No? Good job I asked then, wasn't it?
There are two different procedures. One is for the lengthening and one is for the enlargement. They're usually done at the same time as a day case. It's under a local anaesthetic but with sedation.
Under a local? Goodness me!
Yes, but with sedation, and there's an anaesthetist present.
So what's the length improvement?
It varies from patient to patient but it's somewhere between one and a half to two and a half inches.
Right. Does it work?
Absolutely – we've done over six hundred of them.
No no, I mean does *it* work? Afterwards, you know, the organ, does it continue to work normally?
Oh yes, absolutely.
So how much does it cost?
£3,500.
Ooh, I'm not sure if he can afford that. If he only wanted it lengthened about half an inch, would he get a reduction for that?
Nice idea. Afraid not.
Do you ever get a request for the opposite? That's more likely to be my particular problem, I think – a request for penile shortening. Or does that never happen?
No, never heard of that.
You don't do that one?
No.
Never mind. I'll let my friend know what you've said. Goodbye.
Bye.

So here it is, merry Christmas

Christmas again. Supermarket marketing departments are suggesting, without a hint of irony, that a bottle of olive oil in a wire mesh holder would be the gift of my loved one's dreams. Not sodding likely.

Imagine the surprised and delighted expressions when your family gather round the tree on Christmas morn and unwrap a 9kg box of own-brand washing powder and a bottle of white wine vinegar.

I can hear the steady drip drip drip of money into the pension plans of Noddy Holder, Roy Wood and Greg Lake as their holiday anthems are dusted off for another year.

I wish it could be Christmas every day? No fear. What is it about the holiday season that causes heartsinks, non-copers and even saner patients to fly into a panic?

The surgery will be closed for four whole days. You'd think we were evacuating *en masse* to the warmer climes of the southern hemisphere until the great spring thaw.

Repeat prescription

It's not bad news for everyone, of course. The wilier members of the benzodiazepine addiction society know that they can use the occasion to ask for an extra repeat prescription for their Temazepam from every doctor in the building to tide them over.

Even worse are the cretins who show up in the first week of December with a sprained ankle or a common cold and want it sorted out in time for the Christmas celebrations.

Should I tell them to bugger off because they will get better on their own long before Santa has his reindeer saddled up, or do I prescribe methylcellulose tablets, make a fuss about the amount of extra work GPs have to do to get people fit for their party-going, and drop hints about our favourite patients being those who drop in with a bottle of single malt to boost morale on Christmas Eve?

At least the ritual signing of hundreds of greetings cards to hospital pathology labs and other agencies whose mission statement includes the words 'GP', 'lives' and 'bloody misery' has been dispensed with.

I've had my signature bit-mapped and pre-printed onto a selection of cards bearing cheery images of snow-capped ambulances or red-breasted robins ferrying blood test reports through wintry skies.

Thank you for all your letters and e-mails, which show that you're still reading the column and for the invitations to speak at your postgrad conference, assassinate one of your health visitors, sing at your wedding, or whatever.

What is it about the holiday season that causes heartsinks and non-copers to fly into a panic?

However you get through it, I hope you get at least a couple of days off to enjoy with your family and friends. I hope you don't get called at 3am on New Year's Day by a deputising service or co-op that can't cope and is ready to dump five heartsinks on you.

Too drunk

I hope the kids don't steal the batteries from your auriscope for their Game Boy. I hope you don't get groceries as presents, notification of a formal complaint on Christmas Eve, or too drunk at the practice party. Until next year, then.

Foot spas look set to spark a revival

Perhaps Santa delivered it one Christmas past, or you unwrapped one this time around. You may even have picked one up in the sales. Somewhere in your home you have a foot spa.

You know the thing I mean, the gizmo that vibrates under your tired little piggies at the end of a hard day, massaging your plantar aspects into a bubbling ecstasy. As seen in the Argos catalogue every Christmas and in skips nationwide every January.

Everybody has one – at least everybody who hasn't got around to recycling it via the local Sunday morning car boot sale. It is probably lying in the loft or lurking at the back of the garage with the Rubik cube and the Cabbage Patch doll.

Do you know what I want you to do? I want you to find that foot spa, wipe the dust off and put a nice new plug on it. I want you to view it in an entirely new light.

Plastic contraption

To your untrained eyes it may be nothing more than a hideous plastic contraption designed to bring water, electricity and your toenail beds into close proximity. One bare wire and a skull-cap short of an electric chair.

That's as may be, but in the right hands that foot spa might restore the very spark of life itself to somebody at the edge of the abyss. To a fully qualified rapid-response reflexologist, that foot spa isn't a potentially lethal heartsink fryer. It could turn out to be nothing less than a life-saving defibrillator.

I know this because one of you sent me an e-mail just before Christmas describing events at his local bridge club. One of the older players, excited about the length and strength of his partner's holding, fell to the floor clutching his chest and did the whole myocardial infarction thing.

While the first-aiders were at the top end performing CPR, their attention was distracted by a fellow player – a reflexologist by profession – who immediately removed the victim's shoes and socks and started massaging his feet.

Traditional CPR is a two-man job, and bloody hard work it is too. The relief when the paramedics turned up must have been palpable. Sadly, the story has a tragic ending. They lost their patient, despite skilled use of state-of-the-art equipment.

Victim's balls

But what if the reflexologist had had access to a piece of kit that could have massaged the victim's balls repeatedly at a much higher frequency than is achievable manually, even after years of training? Things may have been very different.

Mark my words, you'll be watching *Casualty* next year and the resuscitation room will echo to cries of: 'We're losing him! Streptokinase! Atropine! Radox!'

That foot spa might restore the very spark of life itself to somebody

I'm going to donate my foot spa to the British Heart Foundation shop on the high street. They have a 'no electrical goods accepted' policy, but once they see the life-saving potential, I'm sure they'll reconsider. Why not drop yours off at your local complementary medical centre or even carry a 'foot spa donor' card in your wallet?

No book can rival school of hard knocks

Regular readers may be shocked to discover that I work in a training practice. I don't actually sully myself with any of that touchy-feely educational nonsense, obviously.

After all, I'm busy berating hapless social workers on the phone, writing splenetic letters to bonehead consultants hell-bent on iatrogenically murdering my patients and drug budget, and ridiculing the pathetic ailments of Essex pondlife, which doesn't leave a lot of room for teaching. Not when you factor in coffee and biscuit time.

But I do speak to the registrars sometimes, and am particularly fond of employing the phrase 'good training case for you' as I fork-lift-truck Mrs Lard's notes, followed by Mrs Lard, into their room. Frankly, this is a punishment they deserve, not least because one recently insulted our practice library by describing it as a 'museum' rather than a cutting-edge educational resource.

Major trauma

This stung us into action – and, I have to admit, he had a point. Some of the books are older than the *Reader's Digests* in the waiting room. *One Hundred Years Of Medical Murder*, circa 1980s, for example, desperately needs serious updating. Others are simply inappropriate.

Why, for example, do we have the definitive textbook on major trauma? Even the most vacuous NHS Direct triage nurse should be able to follow the algorithm for Pissed and Fallen Over of Basildon, given that it involves one long arrow leading all the way to the casualty department.

Some other titles caught my eye. *To Heal Or To Harm?* suggests a radical and welcome reappraisal of the core philosophy of primary care. *Asthma At Your Fingertips* is surely begging the sequel, *Infectious Diseases At Arm's Length*. As for *Invitation To Sociology* – no thanks, I'm washing my hair.

But the winner for arseiest ever title has to be the utterly emetic *Still Small Voice, An Introduction To Pastoral Counselling*, which I was so appalled to discover in our collection that I responded in the only rational manner possible: I urinated over it.

One book in particular brought back terrible memories of my own days as a registrar – the Cardie Bible: Balint's *The Doctor, His Patient And The Illness*. I was forced to read this when I was naive and impressionable, and to this day I suffer traumatic flashbacks of Collusions of Anonymity and all that Apostolic Bollocks.

Updated versions

I'm tempted to write an updated version: *The Doctor, His Patient, The Illness, The Inappropriate Visit Request, The Ensuing Complaint, The Failed Local Resolution, Her Appeal To The Ombudsman And My Resignation From The NHS.* But I think there are far too many pages of earnest and pseudo-learned claptrap around these days. Who reads it? Who writes it? And who cares?

There are too many pages of earnest, pseudo-learned claptrap around

The truth is, I don't really hold with book-learning. No amount of pontificating about the Drug Doctor and Zen mysticism helps me get through a consultation with some whining, polysymptomatic, list-wielding pillock. To cope with this, you need Bedside Attitude, which you get from the Vocational Scheme of Hard Knocks, not from a book.

So next time you're reviewing a book and you suggest it's an essential addition to the primary care bookshelf, bear this in mind: you're talking crap.

Don't blame me for mangled messages

Dear Mrs Lard, Thank you for your recent phone calls and letters, and it was interesting to read your views in the *Evening Echo*. I was sorry to miss your interview on local radio – unfortunately I had to attend a meeting with a representative from my medical defence body.

Let me say straight away that this unfortunate incident would never have occurred had I realised the Government's plan to send patients copies of all correspondence between GPs and consultants had already been implemented.

Medical language

Doctors communicating between themselves tend to use medical language, which is obviously prone to misinterpretation. To answer the specific points you raise:

1. My introductory paragraph to the specialist included the phrase 'Can you take a look, old chap?' – a familiarity borne from the fact that I have known this particular surgeon for years and value his opinion.

Unfortunately, my secretary misheard this on my dictation tape as 'cantankerous old bat'. It should be obvious that this is an error, as you are only 38.

2. For 'is a complete pain in the arse', please substitute 'has' for 'is': a simple typo completely altering what was a technical description of the symptoms of your anal fissure about which you have been particularly stoical.

3. In the third paragraph, the sentence should have read, 'I haven't done a rectal examination'. It was certainly not my intention to say: 'To do a rectal examination on this fat piece of pond life I'd need a glove up to my shoulder and lots of soapy water.'

My only explanation is that my dictaphone batteries were nearly flat and this may have distorted my words.

4. The aberration in the fourth paragraph I can explain by the fact that, with my dictaphone batteries having finally run out, I decided to use our computer's voice recognition software – we strive to be at the cutting edge of technology in our constant attempts to improve our service to patients.

It really is most frustrating that expensive computer technology can mangle the simple message to my colleague 'Peace on earth and regards to your family'. As your GP, I would, of course, piss on you if you were on fire and I'm disappointed that you'd think I might say otherwise.

5. So exhausted are we GPs that it is common for us to fall asleep while doing paperwork. I confess I dozed off after typing your letter and inadvertently leant on the 'delete' key, with the result that 'She is on Adalat Retard' became 'She is a retard', which, I agree, is open to misinterpretation.

As your GP, I would, of course, piss on you if you were on fire

Syringed ears

Complaints offer opportunities to improve our service, so you will be pleased to know that I've syringed my secretary's ears, bought some new batteries, trashed the new computer and intend to get some sleep.

I realise how upsetting this must have been for you and that you might now be suffering post-traumatic stress disorder. If you'd like me to refer you to our in-house counsellor, let me know – I'll do a letter.

Yours, Dr Copperfield.

Hospitals dangerous? Pah!

Hospitals are supposed to be dangerous places. I try and stay away from them as much as I can. Not only are they full of sad people who only want to talk about their operation, their corridors are also stalked by the evil doctors of death.

Pathologists have had a bad press recently because they have been keeping organs after postmortems. The media assume this is part of some justifiable educational programme and have been nothing worse than slightly miffed that we forgot to ask permission from the relatives first.

The truth is that most hospital canteen food is so bland that surgical offcuts are routinely used to make gravy. If you ever wondered why all those pathological specimens you studied looked nothing like their living equivalents, don't blame the formaldehyde. Most of them have been boiled on the top of the stove for a few hours to make stock before they were potted and labelled. Anything to give the *coq au vin* a bit of pep.

I could feel sorry for our white-coated colleagues. They trail up and down through a miasma of pathogenic viruses, trying to force food down that's been sitting on a hotplate for six hours since the cook coughed half a billion MRSA bacteria over it.

Dirty sheets

And if that's not bad enough, they have to stay overnight between the same sheets that the on-call registrar and the theatre sister shared and stained the previous Thursday.

There is, of course, only one medical environment that's even more dangerous. Another place where I will rarely if ever venture. I don't care if research has shown that one hospital in three is a cesspit akin to a First World War trench – compared with most of my patients' houses, they are virtually aseptic.

Idiot's guide

If I'm out of the surgery and a call comes through about a patient close to death in the next street then two things are certain. Firstly, the sufferer will be a piss artist with a common cold. Secondly, he won't be expecting anything more than the standard 'take some ibuprofen and rest up for a day or two' telephone advice. So it's the surprise attack that shows them in their true light.

I'm not going to bump up my mobile phone bill when I can deliver the *Idiot's Guide To The Flu* in person. Until you've felt your feet stick to a hallway carpet, dodged three piles of cat crap on the stairs, pulled a bedroom curtain off the rail and wondered why none of the lights work, you can't call yourself a frontline medic.

Until you've felt your feet stick to a hallway carpet you can't call yourself a frontline medic

Somewhere among the ashtrays, beer cans and bottles of Benylin you'll find an overwrapped dick-head with flu. And an iguana. Beware of them both.

The first one isn't going to like the idea that you aren't going to give him any antibiotics, and as for the scaly one, we've just had our first case of reptile shit-acquired salmonella meningitis. If you are going to eat your dinner off the kitchen floor, better clean it first.

Let them eat cake, and chips

Ask any GP who's trying to hit his MMR target: if there's one thing that the Great British Public knows sod all about, it's risk assessment. We're doing our best to explain that vaccinations are a safer option than catching the wild viral strain and it's all falling on deaf ears.

And we are just so very good at risk assessment ourselves, aren't we? We impose cervical and breast screening on women, but decide that prostate and testicular screening programmes would not be worthwhile, even for men. We have the 'evidence'.

I've been checking out the northern branches of the family tree. I spent some of Saturday morning having breakfast in a supermarket café in Oldham. For the price of a McBreakfast in Basildon, I had a white bread bap a foot wide (that's 30.48cm for *BMJ* readers), smothered in butter and covered with an entire dead pig in a variety of disguises: bacon, pork sausage, black pudding and fried bread.

Cardiovascular risk

Not so much a breakfast, more a cardiovascular risk factor. As was the surrounding atmosphere. They may have stopped folk from smoking at the meat counter, but they can still get through ten Embassy Regals as they mop up the pork fat and ketchup with their crust.

This is real life for thousands of zero-aspiration smokers who inhabit the northern market towns. Table after table of wrinkled faces drawing deeply on cheap fags advertised by humorous quasi-cartoon characters on posters either side of the A62.

Every time I write that we should leave these sad sods to their own devices and move on to areas where we might actually make a difference, the editor gets sacks full of mail from ASH campaigners saying that 70 per cent of smokers want to give up.

I'll admit that seven out of every ten might tell a bloke with a laminated name badge and a clipboard that they want to quit, but then they'll move directly on to the woman in the fag packet uniform and collect a few free samples on their way to the lard counter.

So stop it. Leave them alone. Stop throwing packets of Zyban at them. They know the risks better than we do.

Death threats

They might not get MMR risk–benefit ratios, and for some of them not even the spectre of a few dead rug-rats when the epidemic hits will be able to convince them, but it's their life and their kid. And before I get death threats from Class War, the middle class Marlboro Light and 'single vaccine' crowd in Islington are just as bad.

So stop it, leave them alone. They know the risks better than we do

Who are we to impose? My favourite statistic at the moment comes from Australia, where some states have made cycle helmets compulsory for kids. 'Look at the fall in road traffic accident victims,' they trumpet.

Look again. The body count has fallen, but not as fast as the mileage covered. In real life, the accident risk per mile cycled has risen and kids are avoiding one of the few sources of childhood exercise to survive the era of PlayStation 2. Result? I don't think so.

Patients are making me sick

Look, it's no bloody picnic writing this column, you know. Every week, finding new ways of insulting those snivelling lumps of lard we call patients. Or alienating entire groups of 'professionals' less useful or intellectual or sensible than GPs, without saying 'counsellor'. Or upsetting certain patients with ill-informed and gratuitous comments.

Actually, this last one is pretty easy. All I have to do, for example, is juxtapose the words seasonal, affective and disorder with winter, time and wasters. Cue massive postbag from 'Outraged with SAD'.

I realise that some of you do appreciate my efforts to remain irascible and unreasonable, and I know you also notice the sparkling nugget of truth found at the core of every column – your e-mails and letters tell me.

It is gratifying to know there's a communal pool of bile out there to be spat at whoever deserves it. Patients, mostly.

Absinthe inspiration

But sometimes the inspiration just isn't there. Sometimes I look at my deadline and think: 'Arse. I can't do it. I just don't know another 550 words.' Like now. So, desperately seeking ideas, I've been drinking some of the absinthe Mrs Copperfield kindly gave me for Christmas.

All I can say is, no wonder I'm having trouble writing my column, given the aardvark sitting at my desk reading my copy of *Viz's Crap Jokes*. And it's odd how gravity is working sideways, which must be why I'm stuck to this wall. Ahem. Think I'll go for a little lie down.

That's better. Actually, the problem is less inspiration than perspiration. Because as soon as I start considering my column, I begin to think about the punters. Then I start sweating, shaking and panicking. This also happens every time I anticipate going back to work after a weekend off – my bowels simply won't have it.

I only have to visualise a patient and I'm clammy and palpitating. If I imagine a whole surgery, I'm scrabbling around with carpopedal spasm looking for a brown paper bag. Or absinthe. You try writing a sodding column in that state.

Irrational fear

Anyway, the diagnosis is clear. I have developed an irrational fear resulting in avoidance behaviour. I am suffering from patient phobia and the treatment options are clear.

We could form the Patient Phobic Support Group and try to get compensation for our trauma

One: Flooding therapy, that is to say, confront a whole waiting room of the buggers. No way. Two: Desensitisation – imagine a patient, look at a picture, touch a blow-up rubber doll of Mrs Heartsink and so on. Not bloody likely. Three: Avoid the anxiety-inducing situation. Now you're talking.

Sign me off sick with my patient phobia. Anyone out there care to join me? We could form the Patient Phobic Support Group, rope in some lawyers and try to get compensation from the Government for our trauma.

After all, suffering a reflex vomit whenever a patient says: 'Anyway, that's not why I came,' must be worth a few quid. And if they decide that patient phobia is known in GP circles as 'normality' then sod it, I've got SAD, then.

Put a foot wrong and you're screwed

Oh, sod this for a lark. I've just realised there are now 11 different ways we can get screwed by the system if we put a foot wrong. It was bad enough when I was training. I learned about 'Triple Jeopardy', which ran something like this:

In the days before co-operatives and primary care centres, you got a telephone call at 3am along the lines of: 'My kid has a high fever, stiff neck and a funny rash that doesn't disappear when I press on it with a glass.'

If you didn't visit then you could be up for serious professional misconduct and be in breach of your terms of service whatever happened. But you could also be done for negligence if the child suffered long-term brain damage as a result of a delay in diagnosis. If you visited but missed the diagnosis, it would still have been a breach (failure to refer) and subject to a claim for negligence, but the GMC would be happy. The only way to upset them would be to demand a consolation sexual favour from the mother.

Sexual favour

By the way, even if you examined, diagnosed, treated and transferred the child with life-saving aplomb, the sexual favour rule still applied – even if the mother insisted.

If only life were so simple these days. You and I line up every morning against a full 11-man team of individuals, committees and organisations whose mission statements include the words 'GP', 'life' and 'bleeding misery'.

In goal we have the coroner, who can order an inquest into any death he considers to be inadequately explained. Which is, of course, every death that takes place in a nursing home or at the patient's residence.

You don't really know what it is that carries your patients off, unless you have the syringe in your hand at the time of death, and neither do I.

Go to a few postmortems and you'll soon discover that seven times out of ten even the surgeons who were operating on the deceased hours earlier will still have no clue as to the true cause of death. Smug, clever-clever pathologists have it far too easy, work through much bigger incisions and you never see one with a hungry dog.

Strike force

Across the back four we have practice-based complaints procedures, the independent review panels set up by health authorities, the misuse of drugs tribunal (whatever that is) and the Ombudsman acting as sweeper.

The midfield engine room is the health authority's medical discipline committee, the GMC's performance review panel and the family health services appeal authority.

The team's mission statement includes the words 'GP' and 'bleeding misery'

Up front, you'll find the patient's solicitor playing a deep role behind the strike force of the GMC's professional conduct committee and the Crown Prosecution Service.

Just after the Shipman story broke, I wrote that I was always pleasantly surprised how often patients would accept a simple explanation and apology if things went wrong.

But if the shit does hit the fan – and every time I switch on the television at lunchtime there's an ambulance chaser on the screen touting for business – would it be too much to ask that the GP gets one single fair hearing?

Patients are daft, but I'll tell you about a nurse . . .

It seems patients don't have the franchise on stupidity. True, they are consistently excellent at being moronic, and my delight at yet another example of their intellectual incompetence is matched only by my excitement at wondering how and when this will be trumped. Because it always is.

I thought, for example, that the mum attending for her child's three-year developmental check without the relevant three-year-old had to represent the pinnacle of air-headedness. And yet, two weeks later, one father telephoned my colleague because he was having difficulty interpreting the tumbler test on his spotty toddler.

At the ensuing visit, it rapidly became clear why. Instead of trying to blanch the rash with the tumbler, he was simply peering at it, through the glass, from a distance of about a foot.

Magical appearance

Presumably he was expecting 'THIS IS NOT MENINGITIS, DUMB-ASS' to appear magically.

These stories are true. And they are more credible than the incident that reminded me it's not only patients who have doggy-do's for brains.

We're all familiar with patients being bounced back to us via pre-op assessment clinics with the message: 'The nurse said my blood pressure was too high' – it having been measured once, with a narrow cuff, on a patient with arms the size of Stuart Pearce's thighs, immediately after being told all the possible complications of his aortic aneurysm repair.

This I can take on the chin. But the other day, one particular patient on the rebound from the assessment clinic anxiously explained that the nurse had problems finding her pulse. She had solemnly been told her GP would need to check this.

Think about it. If you can't find a pulse, then you can construct only two hypotheses. One: the patient's pulse is hard to feel, which is usually – as in this case – a matter of lard. And two: the patient is dead.

Difficult diagnosis

Admittedly, death can sometimes be hard to diagnose accurately. In such a situation, I'm an advocate of the diagnostic use of time – I review in a week. By which time they may not smell too good, but at least I can be sure of myself.

But diagnosing life is easier, as there are clear physical signs to help, such as the patient's ability to talk, walk and complain. And the presence of life effectively excludes a diagnosis of death. QED.

The good news is this patient is alive. The bad news is that your nurse is brain-dead

I've made this sound more complicated than it is, and this level of logic should be within the grasp of the average protozoan. So I dictated a quick note to the supervising consultant. 'Re Mrs X,' I said. 'The good news is that this patient is alive. The bad news is that your nurse is brain-dead.'

No shred of evidence in rules

I was feeding some NICE guidelines through the shredder the other day – I thought the CHI police, when they finally come, might look favourably on a ticker-tape welcome – when I was struck by a distressing thought. Not that some earnest, speccy clinical governance git would get wind of the fact that I was making confetti out of guidelines, – but that, one day, GPs will start to take them seriously.

We GPs are in the privileged position of finding it perfectly reasonable to ignore them. After all, anything written by academics which presumes to create order from the chaos that is primary care just has to be bollocks. But this pleasingly cavalier approach will, I fear, change. As I write, a generation of medical students is being brainwashed into believing that patients and their illnesses can be reduced to this algorithm or that care pathway.

I know this because, the other day, a student sat in on my surgery. Bored of playing childish games, like 'Guess What The Next Patient Will Have Wrong With Him And Treat Him For That Anyway' (amazing how you can get a patient with crushing central chest pain to 'try' Anusol), I asked the student my favourite question: What is hypertension?

Snap answer

I expected the usual umms culminating in a look of admiration at the profundity of my inquiry, and a request for me to scatter pearls of wisdom about risk-factor weighting and whole-person medicine.

Instead, I received a snap answer: 140 over 90. No ifs, buts or maybes. Anyone with a BP over this figure is hypertensive and needs treatment. Why? Because the latest guidelines from the Academy of Complete Twats Who've Never Done a Day's General Practice In Their Lives say so.

Flexible thinking

After I'd cuffed him about the head for his impudence, I pointed out the shortcomings of this approach: the medicalisation of a quarter of the population, the perils of iatrogenesis, the need for flexible thinking, the fact that, in ten year's time, we'd be treating nothing but hypertension. And that guidelines are basically cack.

But he was unshakeable. He told me huffily that the guidelines represent an authoritative body of opinion (subtext: you're barking) and he had an exam to pass (subtext: if he fails, he's going to sue me).

To prove I'm not a complete nihilist, I revealed to him my extensive knowledge of the BTS asthma guidelines: blue one, then brown one, then perm one from lots. And send bad ones to hospital. This is the only guideline I've ever followed – because I can remember it, it has no competition, it doesn't change every ten minutes and it correlates with what I did before the guidelines.

I was a bit tired of the cocky sod, so I put him through the shredder, too

But he was unimpressed and, to be blunt, I was a bit tired of the cocky sod by now. So I put him through the shredder, too. OK, this won't help the recruitment crisis, but it'll do wonders for the future NHS drug budget. Now, where are those guidelines on getting blood out of carpets?

A heartsink match made in heaven

Several years ago, we were introduced to the concept of the heartsink patient. Now I think the NHS is ready to face up to and deal with its logical progression, the heart-sink nurse, or HSN.

Whenever a heartsink nurse's initials appear in the margin of a patient's medical record on my desk or in the message book at reception, two things are certain. First, something crap is about to happen, and second, it's probably going to waste several minutes of my valuable *Loaded*-reading time.

'Could you just take a look at . . . ?' will inevitably be an invitation to view something either anatomically normal or mind-numbingly trivial.

Sending heartsink nurses on training courses to try and educate them in an effort to reduce their own doctor-dependent behaviours has proved futile.

Poxy problem

Whenever an HSN returns from a training course in, for example, diabetes, the hapless GP in the firing line will have to spend weeks dealing with mindless bollocks about the diagnosis and management of patients who were, and still are, coping very well with their condition without unwanted interference from medical staff.

Combine the skills of a heartsink nurse with the abilities of a manipulative heartsink patient and you're dealing with forces that no earthly power can control.

'You have to see Mr Scrag tomorrow. He's type 1, not sticking to his diet, not monitoring his blood sugars, not turning up for outpatients and not going along to his educational programme.

'You've got to tell him about the harm he's doing to himself, doctor . . .'

Why me? Why now? You can tell the HSN has just completed a comprehensive training course dealing with every last useless detail about diabetes because she's started saying 'type 1' instead of insulin-dependent.

I know for a fact that Mr Scrag has *never* pricked his finger in his life, despite collecting 40 quid's worth of testing strips every month.

He has absolutely no idea about the long-term risks involved with poor glycaemic control.

Smiley faces

But he has figured out that if he lets his blood sugar ride the hyper/hypo roller-coaster, he wakes up every now and again surrounded by lots of caring smiley faces who haven't yet learnt what an annoying little toe-rag he really is.

But hang on a minute! The last time I suggested nurses got on with doing their job rather than running to the nearest GP every 15 minutes for a quick arse-cover, they went mental.

Sending heartsink nurses on training courses has proved futile

Didn't I know that nurses were much better communicators than doctors?

Hadn't anyone told me that patients remember far more information after a chat with a nurse than they do after a consultation with a GP?

So when I next see Mr Scrag I'm going to lock him in a small sound-proofed room with the nearest HSN.

They deserve each other, will love each other and, best of all, they will keep each other out of my way.

Finding that little bit of quality time

For some reason, I'm popular at the moment. I realise that fashions change and that this bizarre state of affairs is unlikely to last, but as things stand, the next available appointment for a dollop of my wit and wisdom is eight days distant.

I took a week off recently, which wiped out 15 days worth of appointments. Every member of the Heartsink All-Stars booked in for a waste-of-time check-up consultation in the week before I left. Then they all booked another for the week I returned, in case they had fallen ill while I was away.

As they'd made the appointment, even though nothing had happened to them, they thought they had better keep it, especially as they know how difficult it is to get to see me.

That was about a month ago, but the system shows no sign of catching up. If you're breathing your last, I might be able to squeeze you in on Thursday.

Feigning interest

With time in such short supply, I've decided to bring plans 'R' and 'Z' into action. Plan 'R' is the adoption of a 'Get to the bloody point, woman' policy when dealing with nursing and reception staff.

When cornered, I insist that they preface their story with a brief précis and an indication of the total length of time they expect me to spend feigning interest. None of this, 'Have you got a minute, Tony?' stuff in the corridor.

I want detailed proposals along the lines of, 'Tony, can I spend eight minutes and 35 seconds telling you about Mrs Botting's leg ulcer, including an entertaining diversion about a local pig farmer and a film crew from Copenhagen, before securing a repeat prescription?'

Plan 'Z' is the 'Just say yes' policy. I am usually the only person in my profession who shows any aptitude in the use of the word, 'no'. Ask any of my partners to do something, no matter how trivial, and they will agree. Ask me, and 19 weeks out of 20 you'll receive a polite but firm, 'No thank you, I'd rather spend the time reorganising my CD collection.'

The drawback is that this approach often leads into a discussion about the merits of the task, the chance of rewards in the afterlife and enhanced street credibility if I were to rise to the challenge and accept.

Invariably futile

These are invariably futile, but are time-consuming in themselves. Every now and then, I wrong foot the opposition by agreeing to everything they ask.

If you're breathing your last, I might be able to squeeze you in

'Tony, could you write an interim report for the PCG's PMS D&T committee with your LMC R&D hat on?' 'No problem.' Then I do absolutely nothing. When the reminder letter arrives, I reply with gushing enthusiasm and apologise for the delay. Then I forget all about it. By the time I am shredding faxes marked 'URGENT!' and ignoring frantic phone calls eight hours short of the deadline, the victim is usually starting to catch on and is writing the report himself.

Now, do I file Roger Waters' solo version of *The Wall* under 'W' or 'P' for Pink Floyd? It's nice to have time to think these things through.

Political correctness gone too far

A noble literary tradition bites the dust – GPs must no longer write derogatory acronyms in their patients' records.

And so another nail is driven into the coffin labelled 'humour, mischief and pragmatism'.

Po-faced homogeneity is expanding to consume us all, thanks to the domination of the PC world – by which I mean political correctness rather than the computer retailer.

Which makes me realise that maybe there is a point to this anti-acronym finger-wagging, as abbreviations obviously can create ambiguity.

Perhaps I should admit that rudeness in the form of acronyms in the records is completely unacceptable. It's true, insults should be written out in full, or there's the danger that they might be misinterpreted as something innocuous.

Thus, writing 'NFB' could be misconstrued tragically as 'No foreign body' whereas, in fact, my intention is to convey the clear diagnosis, 'Normal for Basildon'. 'SIG' could be mistaken for an abbreviation of sigmoidoscopy; now the scope for confusion has been highlighted, I can see why it's vital to spell out, fully, 'Stupid ignorant git', in flashing neon.

Banana skin

Thank God someone has pointed out this potential banana skin. And who do we have to thank for this guidance? You'll probably be less than stunned to hear that the anti-acronym league is to be found within the MDU.

Just in case you've not come across that one before, that's not 'Makers of Desirable Ukeleles', but, of course, the 'Medical Decerebrate Union'.

I can live with this guidance to a point, but when it's suggested that 'TATT' – a universally recognised acronym for a universally common complaint – should be consigned to the Great Abbreviation Bin then I feel I have to protest.

Not only does 'TATT' save us writing out 'Tired All The Time' which, as we record it a hundred times a week, would make us Very Tired All The Time Indeed (VTATTI), it sounds vaguely pejorative while being quite innocent. Perfect.

TATT is the best acronym in the world, ever. Banning it is like burning art – pointless, destructive and moronic.

Alarmist propaganda

Those who make a living spouting this alarmist propaganda are, in effect, saying that nothing should be truncated or abbreviated in the notes.

This represents another triumph for defensive medicine over common sense. After all, to keep the defence bodies happy, I could write up my notes in illuminated script – a few extra seconds on each consultation for the sake of aesthetic clarity would seem irrelevant to the outsider.

TATT is the best acronym in the world. Banning it is like burning art

But in the pressurised, high throughput world of primary care, these impositions multiply throughout a surgery and can, by the end, add up to a significant delay – the difference between a coffee or thirst. And a tense, rushing, decaffeinated doctor is the biggest medicolegal risk I know.

Does the MDU really want to take the fun and pragmatism out of medicine? Has its common sense gone AWOL? Do I have to spell out what I mean?

The catch-all beauty of syndrome X

It looks as though the chronic fatigue fad has run its course. I haven't seen a new 'case' in ages. What I am looking forward to now is my first consultation about 'Cardiac Syndrome X'.

It is far too close to 1 April to take this sort of stuff seriously but, wow, what a diagnosis! When I was a student, in the days before anyone knew anything about malignant bone marrow, one of the smallest print diseases in my very Short Textbook of Haematology was 'Histiocytosis X'.

At last, a disease that conspiracy theorists everywhere could take to their bosoms. I have absolutely no idea what became of 'Histiocytosis X', but my unmitigated admiration goes to anybody who was honest enough to admit he hadn't a diagnostic clue and who came up with such a spooky name for a mysterious malady.

I don't know what it is about the letter X. Whether it's X-rays, Generation X, X-rated or even X marks the spot, X has something funky about it. I'd have been proud to tell my friends I had Histiocytosis X.

Cast-iron explanation

Cardiac Syndrome X, in case you haven't heard, is the absolute, cast-iron, dog's danglers, scientifically proven, watertight and tax-deductible explanation for those funny sharp chest pains that neurotic 30-somethings get over the left side of their chest.

You don't even need to know the correct treatment is strong painkillers and a healthier lifestyle, because that's almost certainly what you prescribe already, whether you call this complex Tietze's syndrome, Bornholm disease, the Effort Syndrome or plain Bonker's Hysteria. You need to know that Cardiac Syndrome X is a pukka diagnostic term in a professorial cardiology department in London, and it's going to be a boon to harassed GPs.

As soon as we get on message, years of worrying that we don't have a sodding clue about what is wrong with half our patients will be cast into the bottomless pit of history. No more irritable bowels, spastic colons (although to be honest I'll miss that one) or grumbling appendices, just the sure and certain diagnosis of 'Alimentary Syndrome X'.

Fascinating case

Fibrositis, fibromyalgia, and dodgy rheumatics will be rebranded 'Skeletal Syndrome X'. 'Neurological Syndrome X' will explain every symptom presented by every heartsink who's ever had a funny turn. All we'll need then is a few diagnostic subclassifications, preferably annotated in Greek.

Cardiac Syndrome X is a pukka diagnostic term in cardiology

'Dear Dr Copperfield, Thank you for referring this fascinating case to my department. After much deliberation over tea and scones, I feel that her symptomatology probably represents an omega variant of "Rheumatological Syndrome X", formerly classified incorrectly as the beta-kappa-phi form of the Ehlers-Danlos syndrome, type 4.

'There is of course no specific treatment for this condition, but I have advised your patient to stop smoking, eat more fruit and vegetables and to take regular exercise.'

No wonder no one wants to be a GP any more, when being a professor is such a doddle.

Mr Angry should try a day on the gate

To fill what would otherwise be an embarrassing space, this column makes a repeat appearance in *Doctor*'s sister paper, *Hospital Doctor*. For those of you reading *Hospital Doctor*, this is bleedin' obvious, but please don't let that inhibit your reading pleasure.

And those of you enjoying the *Doctor* version: your role is to agree vehemently with the thrust of this article and flood *Hos Doc*'s editor with messages of support. Because the great white-coated god that is consultant Angry has written in suggesting that a burnt out, bitter old bugger like myself, who says nasty things about patients, should not defile their esteemed medical weekly.

Yet most *Doctor* readers seem to relate to this column. I think this dichotomy says something about hospital specialists. I think it says they know sod-all about general practice and the effect it inevitably has on the average psyche. Consider certain facets of primary care. Patients have open access to a free service that some delight in running dry.

Twitch homicidally

How many frequent attenders or over-assertive visit requests for children with earache might it take before the angelic face of the most patient-centred consultant would begin to twitch homicidally?

We have no gatekeeper dutifully filtering out the crud. Presentations are often chaotic, inappropriate and dramatised by media-fuelled anxiety.

If trying to educate, reassure and create order doesn't eventually take its toll, you're not doing it right. And on the odd occasion our patients really are ill, they can't even oblige us with the correct symptoms and signs. Textbooks describe the fully evolved cases seen in hospital rather than the 'feeling a bit iffy for quite some time', presentation with which GPs are so familiar.

That sacred primary care cow, continuity, is a double-edged sword, too. Continuity and heartsinks go together like a river and concrete boots. And holistic care? This simply means that any problem, medical or not, can become *my* problem. Often at 6pm on the Friday before a bank holiday.

Gatekeeping role

So how is it for you hospital chaps? Let's think. My gatekeeping role means I restrict the throughput to probable genuine pathology, and then only when I've framed the presentation into something sensible and digestible. If the patient doesn't meet your personal quality criteria, you can engineer discontinuity of care by making sure your SHO does the outpatient review. And if you decide the problem is outside your remit you can, with a chuckle, bounce it back to me.

Hospital docs know sod-all about general practice and its effect on the psyche

In short, you see patients for tiny snippets of time, at their most medically interesting, then wave farewell. No wonder you don't get fed up with them. Whereas for GPs, familiarity can breed either a useful therapeutic relationship, or, for all but the most saintly, occasional contempt.

So remember this, next time you slate me for having negative feelings towards some punters. What's turned me into being a cynical doc with attitude is the job I do – which spares you the same fate.

How to maintain tsar quality

Congratulations to the Department of Health on another top April Fool's Day prank. This year they persuaded their impossibly naive primary care tsar to tell us that all we need to do to ensure 48-hour access is to organise our time properly.

So, it's not a workload issue after all, and just to prove it, he's going to carry on doing a couple of GP sessions per week to maintain his street credibility.

If that's what the Department wants, who are we to stand in the way of progress? The new method for dealing with the public relies on tried and tested time management techniques.

GPs have what experts call a 'Low Degree of Control' over our workload. To take command we have to clarify our role. This is easy. The next time a patient asks you to do anything that isn't strictly within the terms of service, say, 'No'.

If you can't avoid the task altogether or pass it down to some lower life form such as a social worker or medical student, then stall until the situation changes for the better. The annoying patient with chest pain who insists on an urgent visit may dial 999 or may die. Dumping, delegating and delaying are all recognised and effective time-management techniques.

Absolute minimum

If you have to do something, do it right away, but do nothing more than the absolute minimum. Don't even approach the law of diminishing returns but consider the Pareto doctrine: there are seldom any rewards for going the extra mile and you can consistently achieve an 80 per cent result for 20 per cent of the effort required to complete a task perfectly.

If you are forced to write a referral letter, make it quick and dirty. Consultants might whine about lack of clinical information, absent details of previous investigations, missing drug regimes and life-threatening allergies but whose problem is it if they can't take a decent history? The more you follow the Department's logic, the more the all-purpose, single-handed lock-up shop referral letter, 'Abdominal pain ++ Please see and do the needful', makes perfect sense.

Set up a triage system remembering that most nuisance callers will give up if the phone isn't answered within 12 rings. If you have to spend time in the same room as patients, make it clear how little time you have to deal with them. Do not under any circumstances make them feel welcome or allow them to sit down.

Avoid asking questions, make statements instead. Find out what the unpleasant interruption really wants as quickly as possible and then give it to them. Certificates, antibiotics, sleeping pills, whatever.

Don't develop any skills or talents that might make you appear indispensable

Don't worry unduly about standards, or let the great be the enemy of the adequate. 'Good enough', is good enough, and 'It'll do', certainly will. Above all, don't develop any skills or talents that might make you appear indispensable.

Follow these simple guidelines and the nation will get the primary care workforce it deserves, 30,000 GPs every bit as efficient as I am. Doctors with tsar quality.

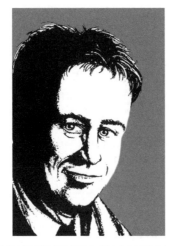

COPPERFIELD CALLING

. . . a
surveillance
company

Hello, are you the surveillance people – bugging devices, that sort of thing?

Yes, that's us.

Great. My name's Dr Copperfield. I'm a GP in Essex. I'm ringing because I think I could do with your help.

What is it exactly you need help with?

Well, I don't know if you're aware of this, but we GPs are having a tough time with patients complaints and increasing litigation.

I am aware of that, it's a terrible problem.

Yes, and I'm starting to think that it might be a good idea to start taping consultations to provide an accurate record of conversations and so on.

I understand.

And I'm wondering how I might be able to do that in the surgery.

There's a variety of ways. You can set up a straightforward concealed tape device in your room. That would be fine for consultations and meetings and things. Or a device could be fitted into your bag – you do carry bags and things on visits, don't you?

Yes, I was wondering how I'd be able to record home visits.

Well, a small device could easily fit into your bag. Or there is a body-worn device that could be worn on your rounds too. The problem with that is that it's a bit bulky and with wires and microphones and things –

Yes, the patients might suspect something.

No, it's just that it picks up a lot of background noise which can spoil the recording.

How small do these gadgets get? Could I stick one in the end of a stethoscope, say?

No, that wouldn't work, I'm afraid.

The other thing is, there are one or two patients who are really litigious. I suspect they're already having discussions with solicitors. Is there any way that some sort of device could be left on their person?

Not really –

You see, as GPs we do various internal examinations and I wondered if I secretly introduced a gadget doing a rectal, say – that's an examination of the tail end – whether this would do the trick?

Er no, you see, these things are too big and they have to be exposed to the air. They don't work if there's too much moisture around.

Well that wouldn't work then. Too much background noise as well. Anyway, thanks for you help. It's been very useful.

You're welcome.

Patients have bugged us for long enough, you see. We really think it's time we bugged them.

Quite.

Therapy for acronym sufferers

One of the great things about meeting my colleagues over a shandy or two is that it provides a forum for sharing ideas, moans, stories and, best of all, prejudices.

It's amazing how enlightening these sessions can be. For example, yesterday evening, I was expounding my Theory of Acronymal Disease to a local GP. This states that any self-diagnosed illness known by an acronym is a recipe for disaster. Consider SAD, ME, RSI, PTSD, ADHD and so on.

I know they are supposed to spell various pathologies but to me they spell something else: trouble. A consultation with a patient presenting with an abbreviation is inevitably long, difficult and bloody.

So sensitised am I to these scenarios that I tend to use a bale-out technique. To the opening gambit of: 'Doctor, I think I've got RSI,' or 'I think my child has ADHD', I respond with: 'I'll have to stop you there, I'm afraid. It's my belief that there is no such thing and if we prolong this discussion we will spend a long time getting nowhere and will both become unhappy, perhaps to the point where we have to resort to violence.

'Either you choose a non-abbreviated illness or I shall have to suggest you seek help from someone more naïve and less time pressured than me.'

Registrar appointment

With that, I put their notes back in the envelope – an act which usually takes a good deal of time and sweat and which has the potential to induce in me RSI, PTSD, ME, or a combination of all three – before adding, 'I believe our registrar has some appointments free.' These tactics are perfectly justifiable. The patient has a choice; the registrar has a chance to see something other than a sore throat; and I survive to consult another day.

Winning theory

My colleague acknowledged this profound insight but then trumped it with a theory of his own. And I have to admit it's an absolute joy – manifestly true and screamingly obvious once pointed out. To explain: consider the word, 'therapy'. Now, append it to other words. So, physiotherapy, occupational therapy, music therapy, art therapy, psychotherapy, and so on.

Can you see a pattern emerging? It's uncanny, isn't it? None of these treatments is any good. As we all know, each is simply a way of buying time or getting punters off our backs. So, put simply, his theory states that appending the word 'therapy' to any management strategy instantly renders that treatment useless.

Either you choose a non-abbreviated illness or seek help from someone more naïve

This is breathtakingly accurate. The only flaw in his argument comes with the realisation that some other useless treatments have somehow escaped the damning 'therapy' tag. To remedy this, I suggest renaming 'counselling' as: 'how does that make you feel, one lump or two? therapy.'

So educational are these conversations that I'm thinking of seeking PGEA approval. And how will this session change my practice? Easy. All patients suffering from an acronym will be sent for therapy. It's no more than they deserve.

What did you say your name was?

I have given up on names, so if the next time we meet I don't immediately remember yours and those of your wife, children and mistress then accept this apology in advance.

I lost the plot with receptionists' names long ago. Like every other NHS practice, we get them young, train them up and then can't afford to pay them enough to hang on to them.

They rebelled against the idea of badges on the grounds that they didn't want to let the man in the street know who they were in case of reprisals.

Now, unless one of them stays around long enough for me to pick up their name by a process of osmosis, they are simply, 'the blonde one who is leaving for a better paid job as a managing director's personal assistant' or 'the redhead who really ought to leave us to pursue a more lucrative career as a lap dancer'.

Sexual Norm

I am not bad at recalling the honourable roll call of our previous registrars, although they are usually indexed by practice nickname rather than anything the vicar might have vocalised over the font.

Dangerous Daphne, Patient-pushover Pete, Bolshy Barry and Sexual Norm have all passed through our hands and left with glowing references making no mention of their acquired epithet or the reasons underlying it.

I no longer know hospital staff below the rank of consultant by name. In the early stages of what I now laughingly refer to as my 'career' in general practice, I knew every medical and surgical on-take team in the county. I had studied with them, drunk beer with them and vomited alongside them in sports pavilions and bars from Ilford to Ipswich.

Admitting patients was never a problem. Any crap about closing to admissions from the houseman and I'd simply inquire whether his SHO was still knobbing that radiographer behind her fiancé's back and whether the SpR still spent all Sunday morning polishing his Toyota Supra. What a shame it would be if someone scratched it in the dead of night during one of my co-op shifts.

Faceless GP

Now I can't blackmail anybody on a one-to-one named person basis, I'm just a faceless GP advising my patients to sue a faceless health authority if their operation gets cancelled for a fourth time.

Worst of all, the only patients whose names I can always remember are the first team players for the Copperfield Heartsink All-Stars, 11 pathetic hangers-on and five substitutes, who stand by in case one of the starting line-up actually falls ill and can't get to Monday morning surgery.

The only patients whose names I can always remember are the heartsinks

So when I read the memo that Mr Bloggs of Bloggs Brothers Bus Company passed away peacefully in his sleep last Tuesday, unlike his 23 passengers who died screaming in terror, I can't put a face to the name.

Until, of course, I ask his wife how he's keeping at her next BP check.

Respect? I'd settle for a rest

It's Monday morning. You've just woken up. And if you're anything like me, your first thought is: 'Arse! – work.'

What is at the root of this lack of enthusiasm, exactly? Poor pay? Professional boredom? Overwork? The comfort of my bed compared to a surgery full of Essex's most viral? I'm really not sure.

The great and the good know, though. Apparently, the reason for our profession's malaise is we're suffering from an acute shortage of respect.

The evidence cited for this seems to boil down to the following, in ascending order of gravity: patients sometimes call us 'love' or 'dear'; they don't turn the television off when we do a home visit; the objects with which they sometimes hit us over the head are getting harder and spikier.

If only patients were more reverential toward their doctors, all this would stop and the doctor–patient relationship would be fluffy again.

Even if I was able to swallow the surreal notion of patients ending consultations Ali G-style with a 'Nuff respec, bro' rather than the standard 'I'll get my antibiotics from another doctor then, you tosser', I have to say I think this notion is utter cobblers. And it's sad how our pissed-off profession has latched onto it so unquestioningly.

Instant gratification

First, respect has to be earned. Solicited respect is, surely, a contradiction in terms.

Second, how can we campaign for something which is intangible and immeasurable? Should patients doff their caps to us? Or would it be more realistic to get them to try urinating in the toilet rather than our lift?

Third, this alleged lack of respect is not GP-specific anyway. The culture of instant gratification and mindset of disaffection means disrespect is standard-issue attitude these days. Everyone is moaning, angry and resentful. It's normal. Let's not be sad enough to take it personally.

Finally, and most importantly, I'm uncertain whether I really want the respect of the punters. This could make life very awkward. I find myself better equipped to shrug off the slings and arrows of general practice life by viewing patients as children, since this is how they tend to behave.

If suddenly subjected to great dollops of respect, then I would have to take their dissatisfaction much more seriously. Though I could face fewer complaints, the shedding of my thick skin might make them hurt that much more.

And if patients start being nice to me, I might actually care that yesterday's case of hyperventilation turned out to be a pulmonary embolus, and that really wouldn't do.

If patients start being nice to me, I might actually care – and that really wouldn't do

I understand that protest marches are being planned. This could be interesting, as participants should march to one beat, singing the same song – whereas the truth is we're all hacked off for different, often ill-defined, reasons.

As the chant goes, what do we want and when do we want it? Er, not respect, not now. Respite, maybe. Resources. A rest from change.

Right now, I'd settle for ten more minutes in bed.

Stupidity is the Great British disease

On quiet news days the editor asks his team of crack journalists to conduct some *vox* *pop* about a burning issue. It works the same way in radio and television.

The difference is that the *pop* whose *vox* is sought by *Doctor* is Great British general practice, and the *pop* whose *vox* is aired on the mass media is the Great British senile demented.

Point a microphone at anybody over the age of 70 and just let the tidal wave of brain-faded bullshit wash over you. It must have been so easy to nip down to the Co-op, lie in wait by the checkouts and get Gladys, 76, to tell the world that she was giving up on buying meat because she was frightened of getting that foot and mouth like her great grandfather did.

American tourists can't tell the difference between foot and mouth and BSE, and are all cancelling their trips to London.

Comedy clothing

Take this opportunity to visit our nation's capital free of fat people in comedy clothing while you can. When we want to entice them back we can order the RAF to spray barbecue sauce over a few cattle pyres in Devon and an irresistible aroma will hit New Jersey within 48 hours.

But back to Gladys. There's only so much that a caring society can do to protect the moronic vulnerable. You can spend years of your life educating patients in the mysteries of medicine and still end up with a troupe of barely sentient simians who can't tell a snotty nose from double pneumonia, let alone foot and mouth from hand, foot and mouth.

No matter how often we tell them that antibiotics don't cure colds, that every headache isn't a migraine or that most moles aren't malignant, they will still roll up to the surgery the following week with another mind-numbingly trivial complaint.

The only change I can see is that, in future, they will be sent to us by NHS Direct, rather than turning up by their accord.

The joke is that the bloke who was supposed to be the one in a billion who had contracted foot and mouth – and who pocketed a healthy cheque courtesy of the *Daily Mail* for his story – turned out not to have the virus after all. He had a decomposing cow explode in his face, and he still didn't catch it.

Blistered genitals

Short of licking the blistered genitals of an infected sheep, it seems pretty well impossible for a human to acquire the virus. For doctors east of Snowdonia, it's a non-problem.

Attempts to educate them just render the Great British bewildered even more confused. Let's get back to the good old days when we told people sod all, labelled prescriptions as 'The Mixture' and enjoyed God-like status.

American tourists can't tell between foot and mouth and BSE

We may have had no idea what was really wrong with anyone and had nothing to offer short of a trip to the local outpatients to consult surgeons with nicknames like 'Butcher' – but at least no one smart enough to figure out that the specimens in the pathology museum were bits of their ancestors could be bothered to bitch about it.

Homoeopaths make me homicidal

The only slight benefit of being on-call is that it inevitably provides material for the column. Of course, you still have to suffer the moans and groans of the malodorous which suddenly become 'urgent' because you can't be too careful, and all the other load of bollocks churned out by the 'how to convert your humdrum symptoms into an emergency' sentence generator possessed by all patients.

Yet today's punters almost didn't oblige. Most of the problems were so appropriate, even for a Sunday, that I found it hard to quibble – although I do think that patients having pneumonia should do so in a room with more than one 30watt light bulb, otherwise how do I know whether or not they're cyanosed? They just look dark.

Harmless virus

Dumb-ass call of the day was for a little girl who'd had a rash for all of 15 minutes. This scared her parents, as it 'might' have been meningitis. Indeed – or dengue fever or typhoid or Ebola or any other serious rash-producing illness which I listed for the parents' benefit to really get them thinking. But I suspect it was just a harmless virus, which I somehow forgot to mention as a possibility.

Then, as close of play loomed, someone obliged. An old lady with carcinoma of the lung – not my patient – was getting increasing back pain. Even on auto-doc, I recognised this as probable secondaries, so I went round to crank up the morphine and mention the word 'radiotherapy'.

A job well done, it seemed, until she said: 'Could you just phone my daughter? – a request which usually spells Big Trouble. I did, and it was.

Having provided a coherent and sympathetic account of the situation, I suddenly found myself having to hold the phone at arm's length. I won't bore you with the details, but the tirade was loud, angry and in essence suggested that GPs are as useful as a plate of cack.

'You doctors just want to fill her with drugs,' she raged. In RCGP parlance, I needed to explore her concerns. In real life, I needed to shut her up, as by now I was feeling pretty pissed off. So I wondered, aloud, if she had any better ideas.

Rational conversation

Big mistake. Apparently, there is more to treating patients than pumping them with medication. Yeah, like communicating with psychopathic relatives. Then, mid-rant about the evils of modern medicine, she blew her cover. 'You don't need to use all these drugs,' she said. 'And I know, because I'm a homoeopath.'

'Ah, I see,' I said. 'If only you'd said so in the first place, then I wouldn't have wasted time trying to have a rational conversation with you. Well, I'm sure your mum will do fine with a few milligrams of tincture of dandelion and burdock. I'll leave her in your healing hands. Must dash, as I have other patients to poison.'

I needed to shut her up, as by now I was feeling pretty pissed off

With that, I slammed down the phone. 'The thing is, your daughter's a homoeopath,' I explained to my slightly shell-shocked-looking patient. 'And I'm homicidal. Probably better if I don't wait for her to arrive.' I rubbed my hands. 'And I do have a column to write.'

Risky business explaining statistics

My next sentence will, I realise, blow my credibility right out of the water. I was reading the *British Journal Of General Practice* the other day. Yes. I know. What the hell is going on?

In my defence, I should point out the following. First, I'd finished *Viz* and *Private Eye* and there was nothing else around. Second, I was reading it undercover to while away a consultation with a particularly tedious lump of lard. (Tip. Do this by placing your chosen journal on your lap, screened from the patient by the desk-side, and assume a downward-looking, thoughtful expression – in other words, the same method you employed for reading porno mags during RE when you were 15. Say 'Hmmm' every 30 seconds and you'll find that, at some point in the future, the patient will have disappeared and you can buzz for the next one).

Patient's willingness

And third, the article was rather good, as it vindicated a tactic I've been using very successfully for some time. It analysed how, in the right hands, statistical information can be moulded to alter perceptions of risk – and, as a result, a patient's willingness to swallow gobfuls of pills.

Excellent. My attitude-based medicine is now evidence-based too. When I want to avoid prescribing punters pills for high blood pressure, which is virtually always, I don't tell them that I'm reducing their risk of having a stroke by 45 per cent.

Dear me, no. I tell them that I'd have to treat 35 patients for 25 years, yes 25 years, to prevent just one punter going a bit weak and dribbly down one side – same stats, different angle. Then I ask: 'So do you want these potentially toxic and nasty-tasting large, difficult-to-swallow pills which you'll have to take for the rest of your life as a daily reminder of this "risk" I've uncovered, or not?' with an expression on my face which states quite clearly, 'Because you're an arsehole if you do'. Don't say I don't involve my patients in decision-making.

But we should take this a step further. Patients' attitudes to treatment should be established before, not after, taking the blood pressure – if they won't want treatment anyway, there's no point measuring it.

Never take

And my experience tells me that NNT stands for 'never never take' as much as 'numbers needed to treat'. Conclusion? We should give up taking blood pressures; an argument I've made before, I believe, but previously out of spite rather than logic.

As soon as I find a reason to stop one activity, Mr Blair finds me another

Of course, as soon as I find a reason to stop one activity, Mr Blair finds me another. Which is why, even as I write, there is a scrum of men outside, hammering on my door to get a PSA blood test.

If you think blood pressure is complex, then explaining the pros and cons of PSA testing is like trying to explain Fermat's last theorem to people who have trouble knowing how many 'r's there are in 'moron'. Which is why I've devised a helpful PSA patient leaflet for them to read at leisure before making an informed decision. It says, 'Forget it'.

Have you got the Right Stuff?

Scott, Virgil, Alan, Gordon and John. Depending on your age, they're either the boys from *Thunderbirds*, or they're the Mercury astronauts who pioneered the US space programme. Either way, they had ample portions of the Right Stuff.

GPs have the Right Stuff too, and need to draw on every last ounce of our reserves to cope in a world where even our dumbest patients recognise we are overworked.

A couple of weeks ago I read about a classmate from my old school, who, as well as working as a full-time GP, is doing clever computer network things to make signing repeat prescriptions a thing of the past. He has the Right Stuff.

I pounced on a headline 'Nurse shortage worsens', and noticed the obligatory 'obviously doing his best' photo of a GP who has to offer nurses £30,000 a year to attract them to his inner-city location.

Visible in the background was a copy of *Snell's Clinical Anatomy* – identical to the edition on my own bookshelf.

School buddies

He and I were medical school buddies and I still have the watch he bought me for my twenty-first birthday.

He works in Pimlico, and nurses who join him have to fork out for season tickets into SW1 from the parts of town where they can afford to live. Last I heard of him he was working in High Wycombe, so he's obviously got the Right Stuff to move upmarket.

Another headline, 'Nurses could become doctors' sent a shiver down my spine. It seems the NHS is to set up its own version of the Open University, allowing staff to work for additional qualifications.

I confess that I once encouraged a staff nurse to apply for a place at medical school. In mitigation I plead that (a) she had a body to die for and (b) she had only ended up in nursing because she had lost her medical school place at the end of her first year in circumstances too awful to document in public. She is now a GP, and one of the best. She has the Right Stuff.

Study hours

Doctors are not made, they are born, and you either have enough of the Right Stuff to be one – in which case you will put in the hours of study during your teenage years when your peer group is out on the piss – or you don't, in which case you end up training to be a dentist, pharmacist, or worse still, at a polytechnic on a degree course to become a nurse practitioner.

Doctors are not made, they are born, and you either have enough of the Right Stuff, or you don't

Dentists and pharmacists stick at their jobs. Like ours, their set-up means they have financial incentives to minimise time off sick.

Nurses, on the other hand, seem to lack that certain something. A recent study from Finland showed senior nurses took three times more sick leave than doctors, despite identical patterns of illness, health outcomes and self-perceived health status.

You can try to disguise the differences all you like, but you won't fool anybody. Being a doctor goes much further than skin deep.

'Tony, there's a man outside with a bill.' 'Nonsense, it must be a duck with a hat on.'

Pants or prescriptions for profundity

I'm not usually one for philosophising. The deepest thoughts I have normally focus on whether or not anyone will realise I've worn the same shirt for two days in a row and, if so, will this distract them from realising that I've worn the same underpants for three?

Yet, the other day, the juxtaposition of three FP10s I signed during the usually decerebrate activity that is repeat prescribing, prompted a profound insight.

Scrip one: a statin for a 91-year-old. Scrip two: an aspololatinaprilitratedipine cocktail for an 85-year-old, two weeks post infarct. Script three: an ACEI for a barking dement. The thought I had was this: I don't know what I'm doing. Of course, during a consultation, not knowing what I'm doing —or at least not knowing what I'm dealing with – is normal. And not having a clue what I'm dealing with, but dealing with it authoritatively and efficiently, is the very essence of general practice: bullshit as art and compassion.

Weightier issues

But I'm talking here about broader, weightier issues. What I actually mean is, the medical profession doesn't know what it's doing – it has completely lost the plot. Ask yourself, what is the purpose of medicine, exactly? A tricky, philosophical question, but one which, some years ago, might have had a half-way clear answer. Nowadays, a combination of technological advances, empire building, the vogue for EBM and guidelines, the innovation and persuasion of pharmaceutical companies, slavish adherence to the pontifications of the Great and Good, and the workload-induced sheer knackeredness which dulls the mental processes of clear and free thinkers means that, as a profession, we've lost sight of what we're trying to achieve.

120

As a result everything is pitched towards trying to make the punters live forever – which is why we put nearly dead people on statins and the cerebrally shrivelled on ACEIs. Quantity is everything and quality is irrelevant, largely because no one has the time or energy to stop, think and say: 'Hang on, it seems our medical philosophy amounts to a plate of poo.'

Unpleasant pathology

If we prevent cardiovascular disease in the elderly, aren't we simply ushering in some other, probably more unpleasant, pathology? People have to die of something. Perhaps we're afraid to face the tough question, though, personally, I don't think it's that difficult: a quick, thrombotic coup-de-grace at 80 or a festering, lingering death a few years later?

Here's the bottom line. We need a Ministry for Common Sense to grapple with these issues and to dampen the enthusiasm of the moronic, the manic and the mad with liberal squirts of pragmatism. Think how much better life would be if every guideline, every edict, every scare story, every initiative, was filtered through someone with, at one end, a brain and, at the other, feet planted firmly on Planet Earth.

A quick, thrombotic coup-de-grace at 80 or a festering, lingering death?

Until then, I leave you with the profound thought that, the more we know, the stupider we get. And I'm off to change my underpants.

No surrender in patient wars

GPs who write cosily about the doctor–patient relationship live in an environment alien to me – a place in soft focus where they skip hand-in-hand with their patients through fields of corn, stopping only to consolidate their partnership with a little hug.

But until someone straitjackets me in a cardigan, welds a character bow-tie to my neck and superglues some pubes to my chin to compensate for my lack of personality, I'll carry on as normal, thanks. Because, in the real world, it's not an alliance with patients. It's war.

And most of the skirmishes centre on requests for home visits – because, in this situation more than any other, the stakes are high, opinions are polarised and attitudes are entrenched. It boils down to this – the patient wants a visit, and he's not getting one. The furthest I'm prepared to go to see a punter is 24 inches – the distance my finger has to travel to reach the intercom buzzer in my room.

Avoidance tactics

Admittedly, my refusal to comply with the standard visit request of 'get your arse round here, I pay your salary, you know' does sometimes degenerate into some pretty lame avoidance tactics. Take, for example, this recent dialogue:

Patient: 'I'm more short of breath than usual, doc, can you come round? I reckon I need oxygen.'

Me: 'You're absolutely right, you do need oxygen. As indeed we all do, which is why the Government has made it freely available. You'll find it's in the air around you – just try taking bigger breaths.'

Patient: 'No, no, I need more than that, I've had oxygen cylinders before.'

Me: 'I see. Hmmmm. Look, are you upstairs or down?'

Patient: 'Upstairs, but what's that got to do with it?'

Me: 'Well, it may be an altitude thing. Less oxygen at height. Try moving downstairs and give me a ring in a couple of days if you're no better.'

Another five minutes of this and the patient invariably decides he doesn't want a visit. At least, not from me.

Insistent request

Occasionally, though, even the toughest visit refusnik must cave in, but even then there are ways to snatch victory from the jaws of defeat. I know this because of an interaction I came across looking through an old set of records. The GP had received an insistent request to visit a child with croup. He advised the parents to steam up the bathroom while they were waiting for him, and employed the therapeutic use of time, turning up about three hours later.

It boils down to this – the patient wants a visit, and he's not getting one

Unfortunately, so vigorously had they applied his steaming advice that, by the time he arrived, most of the bathroom wallpaper had peeled off. And, as he opened the door to examine the child, a significant portion of the condensation-soaked ceiling came crashing down.

After dishing out some fairly florid verbal abuse, the parents asked him, and I quote: 'What the f**k are you going to do about this?' At which point, according to the records, he offered them some antibiotics. The war goes on, but I'd say that was a battle won.

Deliver us from home birth requests

Three thousand pounds. I know it's a tax-allowable expense but, for Christ's sake, three grand. I could get the entire Scrote family wiped out for not much more than that if I asked around at the pub.

If 36,000 GPs are stumping up, year after year, then the defence organisations must be coining in £100m a year without so much as a no-claims bonus on offer. Honest, chaps, I haven't hurt anyone too badly this year, so how about a five per cent discount for cash?

Small wonder, then, that the sensible ones among us are running a mile from obstetric practice. I don't even do antenatal clinics any more, let alone get involved in the hot water and towels in the kitchen malarkey favoured by the organic tofu-loving members of the Natural Childbirth Trust.

They are openly accusing family doctors of advising women that hospital is the safest place for a routine birth. Damn right, and it's no surprise that the maternity ward chiefs they interviewed unanimously recommended that all women should be delivered at home in the absence of complications.

Malpractice premiums

Basically, the more women we can get to drop their package on the opposition's premises, the lower our malpractice premiums will be.

At present we are well in front, with home birth rates plummeting from a nerve-wracking 33 per cent in the swinging Sixties (before my time, I'm pleased to say) to a much more manageable one per cent by the late 1990s.

When things go wrong, as they invariably did on the odd occasion when I had free run of a labour ward, I want a career grade OBGYN or midwife to carry the can. Remember that the Earth Mothers are the ones most likely to kick up a fuss when things go tits up. One particularly stroppy one, who shared her story with the Sisterhood through Radio Four's *Women's Hour* the other day, was deeply miffed when the on-call registrar caught sight of her CTG tracing, happened to notice some terrifyingly steep post-contraction dips and whizzed her off to theatre for an emergency Caesarean section without so much as a group hug.

Quiet chinwag

'We might as well not have been in the same room,' she bleated. Quite right too. You could have faxed the tracing to him in the local pub and he'd have made the same decision. What did she expect him to do? Sit down and have a quiet chinwag about the weather before gently broaching the topic of how she thought she'd cope in bereavement counselling?

She knew of one woman who had had a rapid 'foetus out of the sunroof' experience at the hands of the medical profession, who had divorced her husband two years later. Cause and effect, naturally.

The Earth Mothers are the ones most likely to kick up a fuss

Let's face it, I don't really want many of my patients to reproduce, and if those billions of little chlamydial bugs are still doing their stuff in the fallopian tubes of East London and Essex, I probably won't have too much to worry about.

If it is inevitable, like death, I'm not frightened of it. I just don't want to be there when it happens.

Medical molehill to money mountain

There's never a good time for the red mist to descend. And driving to work, about 50 yards from a zebra crossing favoured by shuffling septuagenarians is probably a particularly bad time.

The cause was an item on the radio: a 'victim' of some perceived medical cock-up was regurgitating the usual pious rubbish about his complaint not being a route to compensation, but a catalyst to ensure an 'explanation', and an assurance that this must 'never happen again'. Red mist. Inattention. Screeching brakes.

My next thought, as I ploughed towards the cluster of wrinklies transfixed in terror on the crossing was, 'Hey, this is going to be a real test of our practice's proactive anti-osteoporosis policy'. Closely followed by 'how much is this likely to cost me in compensation payouts'?

Atrial fibrillation

Nothing, thankfully, as I swerved and missed, though I probably added a few ectopics to their collective atrial fibrillation.

Some people, of course, deserve their compensation, but there are many who don't and a huge number who hide their motives behind a litany of self-righteous bollocks.

I do wish the media would stop lapping up this rubbish and instead ask the questions I'm gagging to hear. Like, if it's simply an explanation they're after, would they accept a beautifully framed dissertation outlining the circumstances behind the junior hospital doctor's 'error', because even the most illiterate SHO should be able to churn out 500 words on excessive workload, sleep deprivation, too much responsibility and inadequate supervision?

126

And if 'the money isn't the point', can they confirm they'll be donating their compensation to charity, then?

A solution might be to switch off my radio on the way to work. But this just delays the inevitable. GPs know that at every surgery the odds are we'll encounter the compensation culture: patients magnifying a trivial incident into physical or psychological trauma.

My most memorable example was a woman who complained of persistent headaches after a small tin of sweetcorn rolled off a supermarket shelf and hit her on the head. Had it been an industrial-sized vat of pickled onions, she'd have had my sympathy, but it wasn't, so she didn't.

Exaggerated grimaces

On the very day of the zebra crossing incident, I saw a punter with 'whiplash' who, between exaggerated grimaces, cheerfully explained how he intended to screw the system for every penny he could and then had the cheek to whine about the recent hike in his insurance premiums – not a bright idea, as I had my hands around his neck at the time (assessing muscle tension).

Cheerfully he explained how he intended to screw the system

How have we reached this point? Mostly I blame the Lottery and lawyers. The Lottery for encouraging people to believe 'it could be you' tripping on that paving and getting a nice little earner, reinforcing the idea that financial reward is based on chance as much as graft. And the lawyers, for reasons which are too complex to go into but which may be summarised by saying that, in essence, they're all twats.

Give us the tools and we'll do the job

Those of you who throw your junk mail away unopened might have missed out on a particularly entertaining pile of patronising bullshit that was delivered to your home address in mid-July.

Grandly entitled *A Commitment To Quality, A Quest For Excellence And A Shafting Up The Arse With A Greased Pole*, its only redeeming feature is that, with the help of a scanner, it allows me to produce convincing forgeries of the signatures of Alan Milburn, Liam Donaldson and various eminent clinicians.

According to the introduction, the vast majority of us are 'good doctors' who can occasionally make a mistake, which should be acknowledged as an 'honest failing'. The truth is that most of us are 'average doctors', and while some of us might be good, the normal distribution insists that for every first-class doctor out there, there will be a crap one to even things up.

Nobody who goes around with their eyes open could deny that plenty of iffy GPs are out there, keeping their heads down, referring everything that isn't a sore throat to a specialist and prescribing whatever antibiotic the last drug rep in their room told them was good.

As this column also appears in the pages of *Hospital Doctor*, I must add purely for balance, that there is no shortage of consultants of an equally dire standard. Surgeons don't get nicknamed 'Killer' as testament to their ability to impersonate Jerry Lee Lewis.

As the Great Leader travels the land, he is struck by dedication and talent. Just like the Queen, he must believe the entire country enjoys fresh paint and red carpets.

Cutting edge

I don't often get to visit the cutting edge of medical practice, so I can't tell you how things are at the practices inspected by the Millbank Mafia, but I do get patients moving into my practice who have regularly been taking useless and occasionally dangerous drug combinations that leave me wondering who on earth has been responsible for their previous care.

The politically-correct view is that this chronic and widespread under-performance reflects a lack of funding and training rather than a lack of concern.

It looks to me as though the entire workforce is, frankly, disinterested – from the lowest forms of life (junior hospital doctors, cleaners) through the middle classes (GPs, consultants, senior nurses) and right through to the upper echelons (accountants, trust managers and those comical medico-political figures).

Depending on your point of view, doctors in the NHS are either markedly undervalued and over-stretched or markedly underachieving and oversensitive. Whichever your point of view, campaign hard for a system where we are at least given the tools and time to do the job properly and see what happens.

Nobody with eyes could deny that plenty of iffy GPs are out there

Alternatively, we could bugger off and leave it to those among us who are just too burnt-out to care. If you want a glowing reference to facilitate your career change, complete with the distinguished signature of your choice, my address follows below.

Leave well alone – and treat the sick

A fit but anxious fifty-year-old lady attends A&E because of 'palpitations'. The ECG taken during the episode shows perfect sinus rhythm, so obviously the diagnosis is normality. End of story? Not quite.

In the lottery that is casualty treatment, they hate punters to go away empty-handed. So they would do a cholesterol check, discover it's 6mmol/l, and tell this patient to see her GP straight away for statins. A needless test leading to needless treatment.

So now she's a fit and very anxious fifty-year-old lady, and she's also locked into the idea of controlling her stress-related palpitations with a cholesterol-lowering drug. Try unravelling that little lot without reducing your own life-expectancy.

An isolated incident? I don't think so. Nor do I think that dimwit management is the sole preserve of hospital doctors – although the white coat does give medical madness a veneer of authority that is hard for us in civvies to contradict. No, to be honest, we GPs can be just as crap.

Hands up

Take a woman with intermenstrual and postcoital bleeding who had a normal smear two years ago. Hands up all those who'd take a smear. Ha! Wrong. A smear is a screening test, remember? A test to be performed in the asymptomatic. In the presence of symptoms, as a diagnostic test, it's pants – so leave hers on.

The correct management boils down to pointing the patient in the direction of the nearest colposcope. But a smear wouldn't hurt, would it? Er . . . a patient getting a false negative smear will be falsely reassured and so could ignore continuing symptoms. File that in your revalidation folder under 'Oops'.

130

I'm not trying to be clever. We're all capable of screwing up, and if you picked something other than my pet hates of cholesterol and smears, you could just as easily catch me out. Take my tendency to confuse hyperventilation with a pulmonary embolus, for example – although both do cause breathlessness, and the anxiety caused by having a lungful of blood clot does cloud the issue.

Shit happens

Anyway, the point is this. These days, the emphasis is very much on medical 'mistakes', which I would dismiss with the cogent argument, 'Shit happens.' If we could shift scrutiny onto the more common boneheaded interventions, as illustrated above, then we might actually get somewhere.

This isn't an educational issue. It's about doctors being knackered and having information overload, so that they lose sight of what they're doing and why they're doing it.

Most of these cock-ups involve proactive care – so all we have to do is stop interfering. Leave patients alone unless they're really ill. This would do a little harm, but a hell of a lot of good.

Most of these cock-ups involve proactive care – stop interfering

I've said that before, but no one is listening because you're probably too busy checking cholesterols and taking smears.

My approach would reduce iatrogenesis, cost and workload. If it were a drug or screening test, it would be called a miracle. Because it's an attitude, it's called nihilism.

Patients' impatience makes me puke

I was in a good mood, honest. And you would be, too, if you had just received a visit request from someone concerned that his 'cafetière is leaking'. Tricky. Do I send him to a urologist or Starbucks?

So it was with a glint in my eye and a spring in my stethoscope that I buzzed for the next 'emergency'. I scrutinised the plump one-year-old bundle of vitality who beamed at me as he chewed and dribbled over my sphygmomanometer tubing. Already I sensed a cloud edging over my sunny frame of mind.

'And the emergency patient is who, exactly?' I innocently enquired of the mother. 'Oh, him,' she replied, indicating Shiny, Happy Baby. 'And the emergency is . . . ?' 'He vomited. Half an hour ago. While he was having his dinner.'

Tension headache

I felt the first twinges of a tension headache developing, but maintained enough composure to extract a history. This was it: up until half an hour ago, perfectly well; half an hour ago, vomited once; since then, perfectly well.

I went over the story again, in case I was missing something. No, he hadn't been dropped on his head; no, there was no high fever, drowsiness or funny spots; no, he hadn't been caught red-handed with the contents of a bottle marked 'Nasty poison, keep away from dribbly children'. There was sod-all, bar one plate of puke.

I decided to summarise the problem, partly to force home the absurdity of the situation and partly to make sure this wasn't just a bad dream.

'So,' I said, 'What we have here is a manifestly well baby who vomited once, half-an-hour ago, and who you brought immediately to the doctor?' She nodded enthusiastically, and I waited for her to say, 'You can't be too careful.'

'You can't be too careful,' she said. I kindly tried to explain how it was impossible to provide a precise diagnosis in this situation, how illnesses reveal themselves given time, how we have to deal with a bit of uncertainty, how attending in such a Pavlovian manner really doesn't achieve much, and so on – not easy with clenched fists and masseters.

'So you're saying you don't know what's wrong,' she said, as to an imbecile. 'I'll take him to the hospital, then.'

Tactical uncertainty

And there you have it. In the public's opinion, inevitable or tactical uncertainty is ignorance, and cannot be tolerated.

He vomited. Half an hour ago. While he was having his dinner

This is something we shall have to get used to. Because, although this example was extreme, plans to meet 48-hour targets for appointments mean that the GP's greatest ally – the passage of time – will be seriously undermined.

No more self-resolution. No more seeing symptoms when they might add up to something.

As a result, we will inevitably over-investigate, over-treat and over-refer, all of which represent new, expensive and dangerous ways to buy time and avoid criticism.

The thought of such a future fills me with nausea, which probably explains why I've just thrown up over today's box of records. Or it could be a virus. It's hard to be sure.

No bed of feathers in a cuckoo's nest

What's all this about doctors over-using anti-psychotic medication in nursing homes? Don't people realise that if we didn't give the nursing staff regular doses of olanzapine they would realise what a crap job they had and move on to pastures new?

As for the residents, there really is no cause for concern. There is no way you can damage elderly psychiatric patients – I speak with some authority on this subject.

Long ago I held down a job as a psychiatric SHO. My job description, although unwritten, was unambiguous. Show up at outpatient clinics, turn up on time for ward rounds, lock the doors of the 'acutely disturbed' units behind me and empty the long-stay wards in anticipation of care in the community. On every count, especially the last, I failed dismally.

Bizarre change

When nice old dears cross the line between sane and deranged, they simultaneously undergo a bizarre metamorphosis from fluffy and fragile carbon-based life forms to silicon-based aliens with the recuperative powers of Captain Scarlet and the Mysterons.

Unhinged single-toothed octogenarians on long-term anti-psychotics laugh in the face of mortal danger. In fact, they laugh at pretty well everything. Pandemics that wipe out sensible middle-aged folk seem to leave them entirely untouched.

It doesn't matter whether you wade in with high-dose antibiotics, withhold treatment or leave things to chance by prescribing oxytetracycline and hoping for a 'get well' card to tip the scales in their favour. After four days of immobility, 48 hours of Cheyne-Stokes respiration and two doses of the last rites, they will wake up as right as ninepence, chuck their bedpan contents at the nearest uniformed target and scream the place down until they get a Capstan Full Strength.

Recently I reviewed a 97-year-old who had removed the elderly mentally infirm unit's full-sized NICAM stereo TV from its security mountings and held it triumphally aloft in a perfect weightlifter's stance before losing his grip, allowing its full weight to impact against the bridge of his nose.

Unlike you or I, who would have sustained injuries too terrible to list and regained consciousness in an intensive care unit hundreds of miles away from home, he escaped with a small inverted V-shaped laceration between the eyes.

Mental torment

If what can't be cured must be endured, in a similar vein what can't be controlled must be contained. Those quirky little behaviour patterns that were so endearing when Mrs Scrag first moved into the EMI unit soon became a communal pain in the arse. Expression of mental torment through art is all very well, but nobody welcomed her reconstruction of an IRA hunger striker's dirty protest in the sluice.

Quirky behaviour soon becomes a communal pain in the arse

Whenever the psychogeriatrician is called in to help, she just shrugs and recommends the unlicensed use of low-dose anti-psychotics for behaviour control. I sign the prescriptions, carry the can and appear as the bad guy when the *Daily Mail* starts a 'free the drugged-up grannies' campaign.

Presents bode ill for the future

Hell has frozen over. Or, at least, patients have started being nice to me. This is obviously a very alarming development. I've checked in the mirror and, nope, I'm not sprouting facial hair and a touchy-feely, clappy-happy expression – I still look like someone who Just Says No to requests for reflex empathy or antibiotics. So it must be the punters who have changed, and that can only mean something very bad is about to happen.

It started innocently enough, with a young lady bringing me a bag of jelly babies as a thank-you. What had I done to deserve such largesse? I'd got her pregnant, that's what. Not through a Very Personal Medical Services Pilot; just the judicious use of clomiphene.

'Why jelly babies?' I asked her. 'Symbolic,' she explained, as she handed over the bumper pack of 50, which I hope was not an oblique reference to the risk of multiple pregnancy. 'And everyone likes them.' Which was sweet, if understated.

Later, in the same surgery, I received the most extraordinary praise from a chap I'd sent to hospital two weeks previously with an infarct. My role had amounted to giving him some analgesia and an aspirin to chew, and praying he didn't arrest before the ambulance arrived – at my age and level of slobbery, performing solo CPR puts me in as much danger as the patient.

Life saver

But, as far as he was concerned, I'd saved his life. 'Think nothing of it,' I said, graciously, making a mental note to send him, just before Christmas, Copperfield's Patented Gratitude-to-Alcohol Conversion Device, which translates thanks into units ranging from 'thanks anyway' (a Babycham) to 'I owe you my life'(a vineyard in St Emilion).

Extraordinary gift

Then today, I received an extraordinary and unprecedented gift. At the end of morning surgery, a little old lady regular delved into her plastic carrier bag and produced . . . a pack of sandwiches.

'For your lunch,' she said, explaining that she often saw me looking hassled and hungry in the local bakery at lunchtime. I was virtually in tears – yes, I admit, because I was touched, but also because the sandwiches contained tomato, which I hate.

Experience tells us that, for every bouquet, there's at least ten brickbats

All of which has left me depressed and edgy. There is only one rational explanation for this sudden and unsolicited outpouring of gratitude: the patients know something I don't, and these thoughtful and appreciative acts have been tokens of sympathy preparing me for the worst.

After all, experience tells us that, for every bouquet, there's at least ten brickbats. So, somewhere out there, stuck in some long procedural pipeline, is the mother of all complaints – and it's heading my way.

And there's probably a medicolegal bullet out there with your GMC number on it, too.

It's depressing that our careers are so fragile these days, since complaints have joined death and taxes as life's certainties. All we can do is fret and wait. And eat jelly babies.

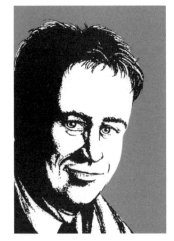

COPPERFIELD CALLING

. . . *London Zoo*

Hello, London Zoo, curator's office.

Hello, my name's Dr Copperfield, I'm a GP in Essex. I wonder if you can help. I'm trying to set up relaxation classes for my patients who are suffering tension and stress. There's been some research showing that looking after a pet lowers tension levels in patients. We were wondering whether we could set up some scheme where we rent out some of your animals for a clinic session in our practice – or even for patients to look after the animals for a period of time.

I see.

Not actually to adopt them, just to sort of borrow them. To reduce stress.

It's very unlikely, I would think. All our animals are screened for diseases and they have to spend time in our animal hospital whenever they've spent time outside the zoo.

That's a shame. I mean, we've done the obvious and approached Battersea Dog's Home and had a very positive response there, but –

We have a children's zoo where there are more friendly – if you like – pets and things, I could put you through to them.

Well, OK, but in terms of anything more exotic – say things like llamas then, or ostriches – then it's just hopeless, is it? We wouldn't be able to do that?

No . . .

Or snakes. We were wondering about doing some research into whether patients we call Heartsinks might do better with pythons than Labradors, for example.

We can't help ourselves, I'm afraid. We have three hundred snakes only. They have a great problem with salmonella when they're handled by the public.

Pity. Have you helped out with this sort of project before?

Not exactly in those terms. We do use some of our animals in hypnotherapy –

Really? Which ones?

Spiders, for arachnophobia, and some reptiles . . . and I know we've done the odd encounter with a mouse or a rat. . . .

The other alternative, I suppose, is I could book for a coach load of my patients to come up to the zoo if I can't bring the animals to them. Bring the patients to the animals.

Yes, that's right.

Of course, I'd want to leave them with you though. Thanks for your help. Bye.

Bye.

Alternative therapies have their uses

Was it Confucius who first said, 'The Man who would speak with the penguin should be prepared to discuss wet fish?' Or was it Eric Cantona? It doesn't matter: the point of my argument is that anybody who shambles in expecting to talk about anything but the scientifically proven is in for a hard time.

I use the scientifically proven to piss off lots of regular punters, too. 'Your kid's had earache all night and I don't give a monkey's' is a perfectly defensible position in light of all the evidence proving that prescription-only medicines do sod all to help.

But back to the plot. One of my partners has been fobbing his heartsinks off with liberal doses of dubiously based para-therapeutic bullshit. His first foray was into acupuncture and moxibustion, which gave him an excuse to thread red-hot needles into the crapulent, yielding flesh of the Lard family.

Malodorous patients

I wish I'd thought of it myself, but the thrill of sticking steel into the enemy would quickly wear thin, as it involved sharing consulting room space with malodorous patients and their relatives.

I suggested he might invest in a voodoo doll and perform the procedure over the phone, but he switched allegiances to homoeopathy and since then has prescribed placebo doses of poisons with his tongue implanted in his cheek to anybody who was dumb enough to take them. Harmless fun and cheaper than citalopram.

Which was fine until he went on holiday. If you thought I was going to spend my summer afternoons handwriting scrips for multiply diluted house dust mite droppings, you're mistaken. Our computer system will issue automatic repeat prescriptions for a limited range of homoeopathic garbage at the touch of a button, so everybody asking for a repeat prescription got a hundred pulsatilla tablets to be taken as directed.

Sorted. Or so I thought. The local pharmacist rang up with a full blown panic attack. Didn't I know that there were different strengths of pulsatilla tablets? How the hell can there be different strengths of a homoeopathic medicine, which, by its very nature, can have no active ingredient in it at all?

Drooling halfwits

He wasn't pleased to learn that I didn't give a flying flick what dose he gave, so long as he made sure none of the drooling halfwits besieging his counter returned to the surgery before the absent partner.

Driving past the local quack remedy centre, I noticed a 'Today's Specials'-style blackboard stating: 'This week's featured therapy is: crystal healing with Dayvid and Karoline'. Why has the deliberate misspelling of a Christian name never featured in the diagnostic guidelines for mental illness where it belongs?

I use the scientifically proven to piss off regular punters

'This week's featured therapy is ECT . . .' I can see it now scribbled onto a flip-chart in my reception area. And the first candidate for treatment is the nurse who has just phoned me to ask whether I can prescribe Adalat LA to her patients in liquid form because the tablets are so difficult to crush.

You point the finger, I'll hurl the abuse

This column has many functions. It fills what would otherwise be an embarrassing space. It swells the Copperfield coffers – though not by as much as you might imagine, particularly after tax. (Any of you feeling strongly enough to suggest that I should receive more might want to take note of the editor's e-mail address listed in this paper.)

But, most of all, it provides the opportunity to gob bile at people who, in my view, deserve to have bile gobbed at them. And there are many. The hit list has included counsellors, teachers, lawyers, private patients, screening enthusiasts, hospital doctors, occupational therapists, physios, the MDU, dentists, media doctors, NHS Direct, complementary therapists, the college rag and, of course, patients of any hue, religious denomination, shape or size.

There are a few old targets I haven't mentioned, too, for reasons too complex and delicate to go into here, but which may well require a relabelling of this column 'A week in the life of a struck-off doctor'.

Justified venom

In my view, all the venom has been justified. Quite apart from suffering the drip-drip torture of patients, the GP has to network with an extraordinary number of agencies, all of which seem to conspire to make the job as exhausting, frustrating and bureaucratic as possible. So I see myself as the cipher through which the coffee break moans and groans of the nation's GPs find a voice.

The problem is, I've run out of people to slag off. Some I've returned to time and time again, because they deserve it. Counsellors, for example. But the torrent of likely candidates for moan of the week has dwindled to a trickle and I fear my work is nearly done.

After all, there's no point in having a pop at soft, small targets. What am I going to say? Pharmacists – huh. Doctor wannabees expert in reverse triage, whereby they send snotty-nosed toddlers for urgent appointments and dish out emulsion of aniseed to infarcts?

Health visitors – hah. Nurses without a uniform or a role, who hope that drinking vatfuls of coffee might dissolve the adhesions gluing arse to chair?

Unfair comment

It's unfair, it reeks of bottom-of-the-barrel scraping and it doesn't really work.

So I need your help. Send me your nominations for people, patients or institutions who deserve roughing up, and why. I guarantee to name the top five and, on your behalf, gratuitously berate and offend each one.

Although it suddenly occurs to me that I've not yet done opticians. They're twats, aren't they? Always sending illegible letters making their concerns completely unclear and leaving us clueless as to what they've told the patient, so we don't know whether to refer, ignore or anticipate an appointment.

I see myself as the cipher through which GPs' moans find a voice

And they're always seeing 'signs of' hypertension or diabetes in their customers' eyes. Result? Anxiety, appointment, reassurance, wasted time. Why can't they learn to take blood pressure or dipstick a urine? Pillocks. Even a pharmacist or health visitor could do that.

Excuses difficult to stomach

They're a funny lot up north. Our wonderful NHS management persuades famous foodie Loyd Grossman to devise tasty new recipes for their hospital canteens and what thanks do they get from the people of Preston? Absolutely none.

When presented with menus featuring 'shin of beef with horse-radish risotto' and 'navarin of lamb with couscous and grilled vegetables', most of them asked what the hell 'couscous' was and told the kitchen staff where they could stuff their risotto to keep it warm.

Some argue that provision of enjoyable, healthy food forms a vital part of patients' recovery and rehabilitation, either by offering a more varied diet than an elderly patient could obtain at home or by depriving younger ones of the fat-sodden, high-salt, sugar-rich junk they choose to buy from the corner shop instead of walking to the market to get cheaper and healthier alternatives.

If people are what they eat, most of our patients are fast, cheap and difficult to keep down.

On the other hand, food could be viewed as a 'hotel' item because we could, and many GPs do, prescribe calorie supplements to nursing home residents on the NHS in a flagrant breach of ACBS regulations, solely to keep them fed.

'Sidney, for dinner tonight we've got Ensure Plus (chicken, mushroom or asparagus) followed by Ensure Plus (chocolate, coffee or vanilla), or, if you really want to, you can try and force down the lukewarm slop our kitchen can provide on a budget of just over £1 per meal per head.'

I once overheard a senior staff nurse arguing with her manager about the number of baked beans that constitutes a portion in one of the granny-stackers in my practice area. Do the math, guys. Baked beans, 24p per tin; Ensure Plus, £1.56 per TetraPak portion. The beans taste better and a large tin provides two generous helpings.

Chinese banquets

One of the biggest things our patients give up when they enter a hospital or nursing home is the freedom to choose what they eat. They can't nip down to the kebab shop for 'two large chicken shish chilli sauce extra peppers mate' or have Chinese banquets delivered. And in 15 years as a GP, I've never seen a pizza delivery moped parked up outside the old folks' home.

I once overheard a senior staff nurse arguing about the number of baked beans in a portion

Anyone who underestimates the importance of a decent diet should consider the case of an eight-month-old baby girl whose parents caused her untimely death by feeding her only fruit and vegetables.

They were pardoned by a judge who expressed the opinion that he perceived 'no malicious intent' on their part. That might bring it down from murder to manslaughter but, after that, m'lud, you've lost me.

But next time one of us screws up, let's try the 'no malicious intent' line on the GMC.

'I realise, members of the Council, that my prescription of powdered hippo-dung in such a case may be unusual, but I really, really wanted my patient to get better.' Rather you than me, mate.

Test results are testing my patience

Most consultants I can tolerate. OK, they have their little foibles – their obsession with personalised parking spaces, their use of the word 'lesion' when talking to patients, and so on. But they're usually harmless; so long as they acknowledge that, while they know everything, they know it about nothing.

Sometimes, though, they get silly ideas in their heads and then they spoil it for the rest of us.

Consider, for example, the hospital-initiated test copied to the GP. Someone on the consultants' committee of our local district general hospital has decided that we GPs are so bored of pharmaceutical company promos and Department of Health memos that we need to be plagued by a new form of idiotic correspondence. So now we receive copies of all investigations performed on our patients by hospital doctors.

They say that it's 'for information'. But I have too much information already. I don't need any more, especially not meaningless rubbish like this. I have enough trouble interpreting liver function tests with a good history and the *Dullard's Guide To Biochemistry* open in front of me.

Take away the clinical context, then for all the use they are, I might as well plug the figures into this week's lottery. Unsolicited investigations with no background information are a potential disaster. Action will be omitted or duplicated and, either way, bad things will happen – to the patient or, even worse, to me.

I finally snapped this week when I received, in a clinical vacuum, a pile of results for various patients, including MSUs, full blood counts, wound swabs, a CT scan and – wait for it – a two-week-old lumbar puncture, which had been performed on a child with a fever (now that's useful).

I said to myself, 'Enough'. And then I shouted the same thing down the phone to some hapless lackey at the hospital, prefixed with the words, 'I've bloody well had . . .'

'But it's all about good communication,' he wheedled.

'No it isn't,' I replied. 'It's about hospital doctors shirking responsibility. By sending me the results of all their tests, they can shift the blame onto me if they overlook the odd skull fracture.'

He promised to look into it, but by then it was too late. Because, yes, in the following morning's post was an X-ray ordered by the A&E consultant showing a skull fracture.

So what was I meant to do? Phone the punter and say: 'By the way, mate, just in case no one at the hospital mentioned it, you've broken your head – but don't worry, as you're obviously not dead, it doesn't matter now. I'm just phoning you in the spirit of good communication?'

'Enough', I shouted down the phone, prefixed with the words 'I've bloody well had . . .'

Instead, I typed a memo which I now staple to all these unwanted investigation reports, saying (in paraphrase): 'You arranged this test, so you sort it out. Yours, Dr Copperfield.'

If consultants will throw spanners in the works of general practice, they should expect me to lob the odd one back again.

I don't know yet where it has landed or what damage it has done, but no doubt I'll get a copy of the results.

Call me at 3am and I'll call my lawyer

It's official – a good night's sleep is a basic human right. If the European Court can side with a bunch of berks who bought houses in Middlesex without noticing an international airport at the end of the road, then what objection can they have when I lodge my claim for compensation?

'Tony,' you'll be thinking, 'you knew the job entailed nights on call when you took it on. You're even dumber than the morons under the flight path.'

When I took the job on, there was an understanding between the pond life and I that stuff that could wait until the following morning would definitely wait until the following morning.

Over the years, in spite of thousands of posters encouraging patients to THINK TWICE AND BE NICE, which most fail on both counts, my kip has been disturbed by a relentless succession of no-brainer calls.

Trivia mentality

My first example was a woman who woke me at 3.30am asking for the morning-after Pill. I can't recall the exact formation of words but I admit that the gist of my interaction with her was to find out what part of 'morning after' she had found difficult to understand and to tell her how pleased I would be to offer contraception at any time, day or bleedin' night, to ensure that she didn't pass on any of her genes to future vulnerable generations. Or something.

The Government's encouragement of the '24/7 access for trivia' mentality has resulted in our services being reduced to the level of the pizza-delivery boy. NHS Direct and walk-in centres are fine – especially for the knuckle-dragging troupe, who don't care much for continuity of care, as long as they get their antibiotics and sleeping pills – but when it's the GP's phone that rings in the dead of night, we have to answer it.

Years ago, when NHS Direct was embryonic, I had a go at GPs in the pilot area who had re-recorded their answerphone message to direct callers to ring 0845 46 47 and then, after a long pause, quickly rattled off their own phone number in a strange foreign accent.

I have to hand it to you guys, you had it right all along. Like the GP who left a KFC-style bucket of antibiotics in his waiting room.

Heartsink nerds

This was to be used by the pains we now have to refer to as 'expert patients' but who used to be called 'heartsink nerds with Internet access'. That GP is quite simply way ahead of his time.

So, from now on, if any patients try and wake me at night, they will not just be running the gauntlet of the surgery answering machine – which plays up at the best of times – followed by a diversion to a premium-rate voicemail service that tells them all about the advantages of calling NHS Direct. Now, I'll also expect a solicitor's letter, faxed from the offices of Prang, Whiplash, Collar and Claimform, explaining why their right to tell me about their aches and pains at 3am overrides mine to a long and uninterrupted zzzzz.

I'll be seeing them in Strasbourg. I've got legal contacts, you know

Otherwise, I'll be seeing them in Strasbourg. I've got legal contacts, you know.

What will they think of next?

I thought by now I'd be immune to dumb-ass initiatives from the Government. But joining the herd of white elephants which includes NHS Direct and walk-in centres is an idea which has me laughing, crying and retching at the same time.

It's called 'inVision', an extension of NHS Direct, and it allows 50,000 homes in Birmingham to have a live TV link-up with a nurse 24 hours a day, seven days a week.

Don't believe me? Well, it was reported in the news pages of this very organ only a couple of weeks ago, so it must be true. And, the story was accompanied by a truly nauseating promotional picture showing an anxiety-oozing mum putting her hand to her daughter's sweat-oozing brow, with an on-screen empathy-oozing nurse over-seeing the whole wretched scenario. The latter sits there like an NHS sponsored test-card combining compassion, (intertwined fingers and cardy expression) and hi-tech professionalism, (hands-free earphones on – either that or she's listening to her walkman). So much for the retching part.

Pretty graphic

As for laughing, the nurse will apparently use 'pictures, graphics and videos to help the patient'. Brilliant! 'Here's a picture of a paracetamol tablet, which your daughter should take to ease the symptoms of her virus. And if I've got that last bit wrong, here's a picture of an ambulance, which she'll need in about half an hour.'

Graphics? I could be pretty graphic to the majority of out-of-hours callers, and they'd only have to point the camera at two of my fingers. And videos? Well, I understand that videos involving nurses in uniform are already available if you know the right places.

Which leaves me with crying. Because, if you pause to get over the nausea and the hilarity, you pretty soon realise that this kind of project is really quite obscene. We have crumbling hospitals, we have no beds, we have A&E departments which look like refugee camps, we have patients waiting and waiting for cataracts to be taken out and hips to be put in.

PR exercise

So, instead of sorting that little lot out, the Government indulges in some PR exercise to make it look like we have a cutting edge health service.

The truth is that nobody needs a video nurse available on tap, not with all the other ways of accessing the NHS which exist these days. This is simply provision outstripping need in an attempt to indulge the public's desire for instant medical gratification and the politician's need to gloss the over cracks in the service.

We have crumbling hospitals, no beds, A&E departments that look like refugee camps . . . and video nurses on tap

So why not go the whole hog? Forget the TV link-up and simply provide, for each family, a personal nurse to sit in the lounge and answer any medical query as it arises. The punters would love it, and the Government could extend the concept by installing a dietitian in the kitchen, a psycho-sexual counsellor in the bedroom and a gastro-enterologist in the toilet. NHS Direct inVision? NHS Direct invasion, more like. And I, for one, will be battening down the hatches.

No-one likes us – we don't care

The headline above is not just the chant of mindless Millwall followers but the current point of view about us as expressed by the mindless Millwall following when asked for their profound insights by people in anoraks with clipboards outside the supermarket.

In-store, Mrs Craplife is collecting £10 winnings from her last lottery ticket and spending it on 40 fags and three scratchcards. She'll move on to buy the sort of high-fat, high-sugar, multi-additive food substitute she buys every week.

There's no reason why I should care about Mrs Craplife. She's not my patient and the fact she chose to squander her winnings rather than buy some nourishing food for once in her miserable little life ought to be none of my business.

The perhaps surprising revelation is that I do care, and that sense of non-specific free-floating caring is probably all that keeps me turning up at the surgery every morning.

Playing brain-dead

Why do patients think we don't care anymore? Because caring, to many of them, involves us rolling over, playing brain-dead and agreeing to every stupid request they bring along: 'You're nothing like as good as my old doctor. He used to give me (insert name of antibiotic, sleeping pill or opiate) whenever I asked for it.'

I'll bet he never mentioned, even in passing, that you're a shapeless, feckless, bone-idle lump, big enough to be visible from outer space, with no detectable cerebral activity above the brainstem. Of course not, that would be 'uncaring'. The fact that I care enough to spare you the excess morbidity associated with pointless investigations and unthinking prescriptions doesn't impress you at all.

The biggest drawback about being a caring doctor is that some of you care too much. The next routine appointment to see me is in five working days, and it's just the same for everyone else in our overworked suburban practice.

So when patients make a fuss, it's understandable that some doctors stay on after hours to deal with them as 'walking wounded', eating into the time they have available for the genuinely suddenly unwell.

Haphazard slots

GPs can't use the surgeons' tactic of dealing only with the trivial and leaving the complicated stuff on the waiting list. Some are reducing the time they allocate to practical procedures, or squeezing patients into haphazard slots at the beginning and end of diabetic clinics and the like.

If you recognise yourself in any of these behaviour patterns, stop

The insurance forms, test results and referral letters that would normally be dealt with in those slots are stuck in the back of the car and taken home.

If you recognise yourself in any of these maladaptive behaviour patterns, for Christ's sake, stop. If we all sink to the level of providing nothing better than a quick and dirty service, where our priority is to get our patient out of the room as fast as we can so we can get on with the next, things will go tits up, that's for certain.

And when the shit hits the fan and the solicitors' letters regarding compensation claims start to arrive, nobody's going to care about us. You can take that to the bank.

Certify yourself fit to realise a dream

I realise that banging on about being asked to write daft letters and certificates is a bit passé, particularly since the powers-that-be are cutting out all 'unnecessary' paperwork, especially the stuff I rather enjoy because it takes 30 seconds and costs the punter a wad.

But it strikes me patients have discovered the days of GPs autographing their stupid forms are numbered.

So, in a desperate bid to exploit me while I'm still prepared to sign anything to get them out of the room within the statutory ten minutes, they're presenting me with stuff which is manifestly bonkers.

Here are three genuine examples.

First, I had to sign a chit confirming that my patient was still alive, so he could continue to claim some benefit or other. I'm not making this up.

Surreal conversation

We had a nice, surreal conversation which went like this:

Dr C: So, are you, then?

Patient: What?

Dr C: Still alive?

Patient: Yes.

Dr C: (after a pause while I scanned his face with a trained and clinically astute eye, checking for signs of life – in dankest Essex, this can take some time): OK, I'll sign, then.

The second stupid little chit involved a nurse who wanted me to confirm, in writing, that she was fit to do a parachute jump. I have no idea how fit you have to be to do this type of thing. Obviously, you have to be barking, but this was irrelevant as she was presenting me with a 'Fit to jump 2,000 feet out of a small aircraft' form rather than Section papers.

So I signed on the basis that she was, at least, fit relative to what she'd probably be like after the jump.

Third, and most perplexingly, a mother asked me to certify that her child was fit to perform on TV. This was tricky: the child ignored all my questions, had never previously proved his stamina on the playing field and, frankly, looked a bit of a lardy slob. In fact, he spent the whole consultation staring stupidly at me, drooling. But then he was only nine weeks old.

I sighed and signed, pondering the fact that, if other doctors took their form filling-in more seriously, then the truly unfit child would be barred from appearing on telly and we'd all be spared programmes like *Children's Hospital*.

Limited time

What also occurred to me was this: for a limited time at least, our signatures remain sacred and powerful. They can make strange and wonderful things happen, such as life, parachute jumps and TV appearances. We owe it to ourselves to make the most of the remaining opportunities by certifying ourselves fit for all those things we've ever wanted to do.

For a limited time, our signatures remain sacred and powerful

I'll leave you to dream up your own, but I've already drafted mine: 'I confirm that Dr Tony Copperfield is fit to have sex with Nicole Kidman and must do so instantly. Signed, Dr Tony Copperfield (no relation).' Which I will hand over should I bump into her next time she's down Basildon way.

And, yes, I certify that she's fit, too.

Market research gone mad

I opened the wrong door the other day. Instead of finding the practice manager at her computer, I found myself in a room lined with cobweb-laden shelves full of medical texts.

No one had set foot in the place for years. Registrars do all their learning from CD-ROMs.

It brought a nostalgic tear to my eye – all those essential volumes the *BMJ* said had a place in every GP's bookcase. They were right. Most of these books have sat undisturbed on the shelves since they arrived.

A dusty fingertip traced along the shelves of texts sorted by subject and then the endless soft-backed workbooks about hot '90s topics like 'Total Quality Management' and 'Needs Assessments'.

Needs assessments were a way of telling patients what was best for them, but making them think they wanted it all along.

Based on amateur research, all of them told you more about the author – who usually supplied the service or product the patients needed – than about the population whose views they were supposed to reflect.

Example: smoking. Smoking isn't just an entertaining way of getting millions of pounds in taxes out of stupid Northerners and then watching them die before they can claim their pension. Thousands depend on smokers for their livelihood.

Small children

There are the workers who manufacture and promote the product to small children and the health care Fascists whose monthly salary depends on convincing a sceptical public that there is a 'need' for their smoking cessation services.

But in the same way that the Whiskas advert gave you the impression that four out of every five cats prefer it (but never actually stated that), research into smokers' behaviour always suggests that more than half of them want to quit.

This, as anybody who deals with the *lumpenproletariat* daily will tell you, is bollocks.

Response rate

The only way to achieve a positive response rate anywhere near that figure would be to phrase the question along the lines of, 'Would you prefer free advice and help regarding quitting smoking, or a pineapple rammed up your arse?'

Even then, most of them would have to think twice before answering.

Asking people what they think is a waste of effort. Every day, our patients are solicited for their views about organic food and happy poultry.

So don't ask your patients what they think they want, tell them how great the service is they already get

They always answer that they'd be pleased to pay the extra 20p a kilo for meat from a cow slaughtered in the presence of a resident juggler, but when the purse is open, the mechanically recovered meat pies and the eggs laid by battery chickens win every time.

Market research told companies that there was a 'need' for the Sinclair C5, the last 10cc album and an *Avengers* movie when people actually wanted a Ford Mondeo, the Beatles' 'Revolver' and videotapes of the original TV shows.

So don't ask your patients what they think they want or need, tell them how great the service is that they already get. Especially for the pittance they're prepared to pay for it.

Some people will believe anything

One of the fab things about being a GP is the faithful and disarming way in which most patients trust us.

We can prescribe whatever treatment we want and, like some dopey Golden Retriever, they always come bounding back for more cures.

For example, imagine for a moment that you have crushing central chest pain and think you're dying. What does your GP do? He tells you to chew on an aspirin.

Never mind that you're suffering in excruciating agony – if the guy with the stethoscope and concerned expression tells you to pop a pill that wouldn't normally take the edge off a tension headache, you jump to it and gulp it down. After all, he knows what he's doing. Breathing your last? Here, try a paper bag. Having horrendous palpitations? Just stick your head in a bucket of icy water.

These treatments have a scientific basis but the punters don't know that. And they don't care – because, as far as they're concerned, everything we say is gospel.

Cabbage leaves

I even know of one GP who routinely recommends that patients with mastitis treat themselves by putting cabbage leaves in their bras. Or is it broccoli? Anyway, it's green and it's weird. He seriously believes it works but, more amazingly, so do his patients.

This touching gullibility struck me the other day when I saw a patient to discuss the outcome of a referral I'd made to the dermatologist for a peculiar rash on his penis. 'Ah, I see,' I said, authoritatively, as I read the consultant's reply, 'you have Balanitis of Zoon.'

And, as he accepted this unquestioningly, it occurred to me that I could have told him he had Ague of Zorg, or Thark's Fourth Vascularity in C Minor and he'd have been perfectly happy.

In fact, I decided to put his apparently unshakeable faith in me to the test when I recommended treatment for his penile problem. And it seems I was right – you'd have to completely trust your doctor to accept that the standard management of Balanitis of Zoon might involve a strimmer.

Special tuition

This ability to so completely pull the wool over a patient's eyes is, of course, a skill that usually requires years of experience to perfect. So I'm delighted that A&E SHOs at my local hospital are receiving special tuition in this area.

I know this for a fact because I recently received a casualty letter for a patient who'd presented with cough and shortness of breath but who turned out to have a normal chest X-ray. Diagnosis? I quote: 'Pre-radiological pneumonia'. Fantastic! If I say you have pneumonia, you have pneumonia, and if the X-ray fails to show it, that's just because I'm one step ahead of the machine.

It occurred to me that I could have told him he had Ague of Zorg

This really is advanced level bullshit and should act as an example to us all.

I can't wait to try it out on my patients – for example, now I can dish out iron tablets to keep punters with TATT happy, regardless of their FBC results. Because, if they're normal, it's simply pre-haematological anaemia. Of Zoon.

Do GPs give a monkeys about heartsinks?

Surprise! I'm writing this in the firm's time because I have half an hour to spare. Of the nine potential victims who called since lunchtime insisting that they were in need of urgent medical attention, only six have shown up to the emergency clinic.

Is it too much to hope for that the other three have died in transit, succumbing to an overwhelming yeast infection?

I am not dealing with the standard Neanderthal *Heartsink erectus* here. No, these are *Heartsink sapiens*, trying in their own primitive way to work the system. Next thing we know they'll be developing basic language skills.

Closing time

They may be planning to roll up on the stroke of closing time, hoping to avoid the punitive waiting around I impose on healthy punters who turn up claiming to be seriously ill.

They won't try that stunt again after a night wasted watching the Cartoon Network in the local casualty. And they might catch a glimpse of a few truly sick people there, so they can recognise one if they see one in future.

As for my referral letter, I didn't say they had meningitis, just that we can't be too careful.

Sometimes I can fix it so the walking wounded spend at least an hour watching other patients wander in with 30 seconds to spare, be ushered in to me and leave ten minutes later, even if they only wanted a certificate.

Anything to keep the time-wasting cretins who routinely fill my 'urgent' slots stuck to their seats in the waiting room.

Exceptions may be made in cases of severe cystitis, but only for patients who look to be treading a fine line between sanity and incontinence.

Facial scabs

Perhaps word will get around. The woman who has just waited two hours to learn that I don't prescribe topical antivirals for cold sores, left the surgery in the sort of mood that drives people to stand on the back of lorries in car parks yelling, 'Dr Copperfield is a charlatan and a disgrace. He laughs while innocent children with embarrassing facial scabs suffer ridicule from their peers.'

The only mistake she's making is to confuse me with somebody who gives a toss; otherwise she's spot on. I even suggested she ring NHS Direct next time, rather than queue up to see me about trivia, which is a put down I usually reserve only for the most annoying sub-species, *Heartsink superior*.

The only mistake she's making is to confuse me with somebody who gives a toss

Time to go – it's five minutes before closing and someone's wandered in with a baby who 'can't breathe and is burning up'. Smoke inhalation, obviously. Luckily, there's a fire bucket in reception.

Don't let the SODS get you down

Apparently, you can no longer die of old age, which is good news for me now that I've turned 40. I know this, because in the post-Shipman era of dotting 'i's, crossing 't's and covering backs, it's been suggested that 'old age' is no longer acceptable as a cause of death on death certificates.

Intellectually, I can accept this. Patients might die on their 90th birthday but they don't die of it. Old age is simply associated with death, in the same way that my reluctant foray into middle age is associated with an irresistible urge to buy a sports car, dig out all my Smiths albums and immolate anyone who buys me comfy slippers or V-neck jumpers.

If we can get away with 'old age' as a terminal diagnosis then we should be able to claim that people can die, of, say, collecting Barry Manilow CDs or supporting Arsenal too – which, indeed, they could if we had sensible euthanasia laws.

Sod intellect

But sod intellect. 'Old age' on death certificates is fine by me: it's kind, pragmatic and hassle-free.

The only alternative is to come up with a precise diagnosis. This will either mean more postmortem examinations, with all the fuss and trauma that entails, or keeping tabs on the elderly much more closely so you can tell the coroner that, yes, you have seen Mrs Lard within the last decade and that, yes, in retrospect, maybe the way she was clutching her head last time you visited did mean a sub-arachnoid haemorrhage rather than surprise at seeing you. One means more grief for already grieving relatives, which is a bad idea, and the other means me visiting the elderly more, which is even worse.

Another option is to smooth-talk the coroner into accepting a catch-all diagnosis such as 'myocardial infarct'. The problem here is if all deaths from 'old age' suddenly mutate into 'infarcts', the CVS mortality stats will go pear-shaped and we GPs will be beaten about the head with a rolled up NSF for not putting statins in the tap water. This could be circumvented by agreeing on some obscure, non-incriminating diagnosis to replace old age, although a sudden epidemic of fatal dengue fever might arouse suspicion.

Sudden death

The obvious solution is to devise a completely new diagnosis. Let's look at the facts: the elderly do tend to die – if you don't believe me, ask any of your 130-year-old patients what they think. These deaths happen suddenly and they're often a complete mystery. Put this all together and we have Sudden Older-person Death Syndrome. After all, Sudden Infant Death Syndrome and Sudden Adult Death Syndrome are acceptable diagnoses, so why should the wrinklies miss out?

We should be able to claim that people can die of supporting Arsenal

If an individual fits the criteria for SODS – abrupt demise of a geriatric who wasn't supposed to die – then the diagnosis should be valid on a death certificate. OK, we'll have to accept a SODS support group agitating for more research and stiff targets to prevent SODS, but I could live with this. Until I get old.

Dear specialist, you stick to your job and I'll get on with mine

Did you know that more people read this column than read the *BMJ*? That's a sobering thought isn't it? No longer will I harbour ambitions to appear in their 'Personal View', 'Soundings' or 'An Anecdotally Amusing Thing Happened To Me On The Way To The Surgery' sections.

I only receive the GP version of the blue comic as I am considered incapable of grasping the scientific considerations underpinning the really serious research that's published in the consultants' copies.

Who? Little old me? I'd never understand all those complicated chi-squared tables and confidence intervals. You mean standard errors aren't just the mistakes that statisticians make on a regular basis? Oh, explain it to me again please, I'm only a GP after all.

Latest studies

It's probably just as well that more family doctors read these weekly outpourings than peruse the latest cutting-edge studies into the molecular and sub-molecular basis of medicine. We're only GPs and, to quote a GP performing at the *BMJ*'s Christmas party and revue, we know our place.

Overall, it's better that we're kept in the dark. So long as we continue to prescribe the drug recommended by the consultant entertained by the marketing department, we can do little harm.

Still, humble GP that I am, I'd like to offer a particular group of full-time researchers in Edinburgh a little much-needed advice and encouragement. Don't lose heart. You are involved in work of national importance. Just remember, cows are the ones with horns that carry BSE. Sheep are woolly quadrupeds with a proven ability to recognise another sheep when they see one.

The risk assessment team would just like you to make sure you sew the labels on the right way around in future.

I mean, it's bad enough when a surgeon cuts the wrong leg off, even if the bloke in the bed opposite does want to buy the patient's slippers, but it doesn't result in a proposed cull of the majority of the adult population.

However, I don't hold with this 'mostly harmless' GP model. I'm the sort of GP who wants to know why a drug called Pregaday is unlicensed for use in early pregnancy, who writes back to consultants questioning their increasingly bizarre and entirely inappropriate recommendations for drugs in therapeutic groups way outside their range of expertise. Suddenly, my local ENT surgeon is an expert in the pharmacology of the upper gastrointestinal tract. Not.

Suddenly, my local ENT surgeon is an expert in the pharmacology of the gastrointestinal tract

Acidic fumes

If my heartsink's hoarseness really is related to acidic fumes wafting up the oesophagus from his seething gastric cauldron, then that's all I really wanted to know. I can pick up and run with it from there, thanks very much.

I know what PPIs do, how they do it, which ones are licensed for which indication, what their dose response curves look like and what their side-effects might be.

Which puts me five–nil up with only stoppage time remaining. Just long enough to stop the half-baked crap he left the hospital with and start him on something that might actually work.

Let's make a deal, Dr Smart-arse Specialist. You don't sod about with my patients' pharmaceuticals and I won't start washing out their sinuses, OK?

In pursuit of last-minute PGEA

At this time of year I usually realise, to my horror, that I won't have accumulated the requisite number of educational brownie points by April. So it's time for PGEA cramming, which means any course will do, as long as it's local and vaguely relevant.

When I'm really desperate, though, even these rules are ditched, which explains why I once found myself in Wales on 31 March at a one-day conference on 'Advances in Interventional Radiology'.

An immutable criterion is that the course must be unfashionably didactic. In my book, for 'small group', 'interactive' and 'flip-chart', read 'retch', 'gag' and 'puke'. And any speaker who begins a talk by saying: 'You're going to do most of the work' should be kicked to death while we chant: 'How's this for group dynamics?'

But my worst nightmare involves getting embroiled in the type of cardie weekend which ends – and I swear this actually happened – with the bonded 'group' huddled in the middle of a field, then backing slowly away from each other, waving goodbye. I just pray the tossers were encircled by some strategically deposited cowpats.

Talking sense

No, give me old-fashioned lectures – how else would I sleep at these things? So imagine my surprise when, at a recent conference on neurology I was jolted into consciousness by a speaker talking sense, which, for a specialist – and particularly a neurologist – is extra-ordinary.

He described some novel and useful physical signs, such as The Paper Sign, in which patients bring their doctor screeds of magazine articles, Internet print-outs or graphically displayed symptom diaries. Diagnosis: nuts. And The Slipper Sign, in which hospital inpatients wear those oh-so-amusing oversized character slippers. Diagnosis: also nuts – especially if they wear them to follow-up appointments.

But the *pièce de résistance* came with his comment that most neurological examinations in primary care are a waste of time, so we should stop doing them. His explanation? In neurology, the history is everything and the examination is hopelessly subjective. If you line up ten of his colleagues and get them to check a patient's reflexes, not only do you have most of the country's neurologists – so don't try this on a busy road – you also have ten different opinions.

Imagine my surprise when I was jolted into consciousness by a speaker talking sense

Unprecedented – a consultant telling us we can stop doing something rather than berating us to do more or do it better.

Perhaps there are other tasks in medicine we could drop. If so, we could develop a new equilibrium to solve all our workload worries: whenever we take on more work, this has to be balanced by the ditching of some other activity.

Less empathy

For example, an improvement in access should prompt, say, a corresponding decrease in empathy, so I could respond to: 'Thank you for seeing me so soon, doctor,' with: 'Cut the crap, what's up with you?' It's take-home points like these that remind me of the value of postgraduate education.

Let's put a tiger into the NHS's tank

Yet again we are being encouraged to make better use of our valuable time. Every GP I know is trying out new systems that will allow the genuinely sick patient rapid access to medical care and discourage punters with common colds from attending.

Such tactics include:

- 'Talk to your pharmacist' – even though he has received no formal diagnostic training;
- 'Ring NHS Direct' – even if they overestimate the severity of your symptoms and drive you into a blind panic about a simple hang-over (but you'll probably go straight to A&E and not bother us again).

It's been said that if you put a monkey into a white coat, our patients will take more notice of him than of us.

As long as the monkey is giving proper evidence-based advice, why shouldn't they? Monkeys are fun, bouncy, happy-go-lucky creatures who work for peanuts.

GPs are not, although the peanut analogy stands up to examination. But unlike GPs, animals can be trained to work to protocols.

In an effort to conserve nursing manpower, I once tried to procure the services of a duck-billed platypus for our cervical cytology clinic.

Intrepid marsupial

A few months' intensive encouragement and reward could have trained this intrepid marsupial to plunge headlong through the introitus, use his specially adapted front paws to rotate clockwise through 360 degrees while keeping his nose up against the cervix and then to reverse back into the light, finally wiping his bill from right to left on a prepared slide.

A dash of fixative, applied by a chimpanzee attached to a pair of electric cables and a peanut dispenser, and *voila!* – the perfect cervical sample ready for dispatch to the laboratory.

But the health authority refused to grant funding for any research project involving the use of animals – domestic, barnyard or otherwise. This appears to be incredibly shortsighted.

Robust research studies have shown beyond doubt that keeping pets is beneficial to health and reduces overall NHS spend per capita, especially in the elderly.

Little old ladies with cats live much more fulfilled lives than their companion-free counterparts.

In a world with an increasingly ageing population, why has nobody studied the comparative cost-benefits of different types of pet?

Consider the tiger. Admittedly a much more expensive proposition than the domestic cat, but the high initial outlay would soon be recouped from the marked reduction in follow-on health costs.

Less medication

Elderly subjects in the domestic cat-owning group would require less medication in subsequent years than age-matched controls without cats.

Subjects entering the tiger arm of the trial would need no medication at all

But subjects entering the tiger arm of the trial would very quickly require no medication at all.

The subsequent expenses – funerals, floral tributes, death notices – would be sourced from the family or social services budget and once the system had been 'pump-primed', the big cats could then be reused for new cases in the same way that wheelchairs and walking aids are recycled within the Health Authority area.

Some would, naturally, appear for sale at local boot sales or in the small-ads columns of the local free press and enter the grey market, enabling purchase by devoted family members.

In fact, I'd probably get one for use in my own practice.

Determined by the toss of a coin, half the walking wounded get assessed by the duty nurse, the rest are triaged by the practice tiger.

Heads, they lose. Not to mention their arms, legs, genitals . . .

Let's-have-
a-pop poll
puts lawyers
in first place

Regular readers may recall that, some time ago, I complained I was running out of column fodder. I feared I might have to retire from these pages, or at least retread old ground by simply running through my hate-list all over again, starting, obviously, with counsellors.

But your e-mails have come to my rescue, revealing a cluster of new targets that deserve a dose of vitriol. Your helpful suggestions lead me to conclude the following:

(a) There are a lot of pissed off GPs out there;
(b) The sources of our pissed-offness are many and varied;
(c) It seems I have led a relatively sheltered existence.

Fallen foul

I mention the latter because I have to confess I have yet to be seriously aggrieved by dietitians, headmasters, ambulance men, doctors married to nurses, community paediatricians, directors of public health, or cytologists – but, judging by your comments, it can only be a matter of time.

Nor have I yet fallen foul of the Citizens Advice Bureau. Indeed, I've never come across this agency down Basildon way, perhaps because the only sane advice it could give would be to suggest people move elsewhere, so perhaps it's taken its own advice and relocated.

But most of your suggestions would have virtually all GPs nodding in agreement and murmuring thoughtfully: 'Yes, now, they *are* twats.'

So, condemned to eternal fires of hell and damnation are educationalists, social workers, home helps, facilitators, drug companies, people who moan about DNAs, and board members of primary care organisations— and none, in my view, can have any real complaints.

I also identify strongly with those GPs who cited as irksome certain 'trigger phrases' – trigger in the sense that anyone saying them should be shot. Into this category fall people who use the words or phrases 'stakeholder', 'seamless', 'GPs aren't doing enough to . . .' or 'the GP is ideally placed to . . .' – although I agree that the GP is ideally placed to make rude masturbatory gestures to the people who spout this cack.

So who was 'top of the let's-have-a-pop-at' list? I'm embarrassed to reveal that it was our esteemed friends in the legal profession. I find this hard to believe, given the recent lively correspondence in these pages regarding the Copperfield column, which revealed solicitors and lawyers to be, as you'd expect, pragmatic, realistic and droll.

We are the final pathway through which other dysfunctional agencies bugger everything up

And if any are reading: bear in mind that it's simply my duty to convey the results of this poll, so don't sue the messenger. No doubt you're having a good laugh about it already.

And I would like to highlight one final point from this survey. The results reveal that it's an illusion to suggest that GPs work in a team. They don't; they work in a network.

A team is all about individuals functioning together as a slick unit – think Manchester United. A network is all about complex, interlinked systems which foul up regularly – think railways.

Common pathway

GPs who bang on about teamwork had better extract themselves from that group hug and take a good look at what's really going on. We are simply the final common pathway through which scores of other, more dysfunctional professionals and agencies bugger everything up.

This network is ever-expanding, it will overload and overpower us eventually, and we all hate it. I know this because of your e-mails, and I see it as my duty to gob on each and every one of the targets you suggest. Except the lawyers, of course. You're wrong about them.

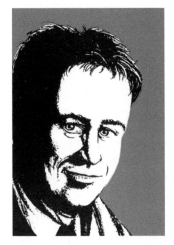

COPPERFIELD CALLING

. . . the vendor of the Royal Yacht Britannia

Hello, Ministry of Defence.

Hello. My name's Dr Copperfield and I want to buy the Royal Yacht Britannia. Can you put me through to the appropriate person?

Yes, one moment please. (A very long pause). Do you know, Dr Copperfield, I've tried every single extension for Britannia and no one is answering their phone.

Perhaps they've all sailed off in her.

Ha ha. Can I take your number and get someone to call you back?

It's OK. I'll try again tomorrow.

* * * * * * *

Hello, Ministry of Defence.

Hello. I want to buy the Royal Yacht Britannia.

Ah – it's Dr Copperfield, isn't it? You rang yesterday. Hold on. I'll just put you through.

Hello.

Hello, my name's Dr Copperfield, I'm a GP in Essex. I wanted to enquire about how I might go about buying the Royal Yacht Britannia.

I see.

What's the situation at present?

The situation at present is that the ship is being decommissioned next year and we'll be looking at bids and so on and then taking it from there.

But no one has a claim on it at present? It's open to offers?

Yes, that's right. You can put an application in writing to the Cabinet Office.

My understanding is that the ship is medically equipped –

It has some medical equipment, that's right. But that will all be gutted in due course.

You see my idea is to turn it into a floating hospital. We GPs in and around London have terrible trouble getting beds for urgent admissions. I thought we could sail it up and down the Thames collecting patients, then treat them on board. To ease the workload for the London hospitals you see. Like the flying doctor in Australia. Only floating.

I don't think that would be possible. It would cost an enormous amount money to kit her out in that way.

Oh, I know a few fundholders who have got some savings put by –

Well just the basic refurbishment will cost millions.

And to turn it into a hospital?

You're talking about an enormous amount of money. Millions and millions.

Oh. Anyway, tell me, what depth water does she require? You see, my local hospital has a river running nearby. Well, more a stream really.

I don't know exactly the depth of water she needs. She's a big vessel. You have to remember that she was originally built as a cross channel ferry. You'd have to dig out huge chunks of the river bed to achieve the sort of thing you're suggesting. She's far too big.

So you think it's a non starter?

I certainly don't think there's any point in talking about floating her up and down the Thames. I just don't think that would be possible. If you had her alongside a hospital or some other facility then maybe she could be used in the way you describe –

So there's a chance –

Yes, if you'd like to send in a formal application. You need to apply to the Cabinet Office.

I might just do that.

Abnormal test result my foot

So what, exactly, is 'abnormal'? I ask because one of my patients who was dumb enough to consult a private 'specialist' about her funny turns – and yes, as any GP reading this will already have gathered, she's as neurotic as a laboratory rat with its genitals connected to a 240V power point – has been told that her *Helicobacter pylori* breath test, obviously a first-line investigation for funny turns in the private sector, was 'borderline abnormal'.

Her specialist recommended an immediate course of *H. pylori* eradication therapy.

The published literature about treating asymptomatic (feeling iffy during *Coronation Street* but being better by the adverts isn't an *H. pylori*-specific symptom in my book) patients with *H. pylori* infections is complex, but the smart money seems to be on the side of leaving things be.

But you know the way things are, combine a positive urea breath test with a neurotic patient and nine days out of ten we'd treat for an easier life.

Unit mistrust

My patient's UBT result was 0.4 of whatever units you're supposed to deal in. The lab's abnormal reference range starts at 5.0. No, that's not a misprint. According to established Harley Street opinion, the 'borderline abnormal range' begins at just less than 10 per cent of the highest normal value.

Or to put it another way, anybody driving on the M25 at 7mph is at risk of receiving a speeding ticket and any man with a penis longer than 1in when fully erect can, and often does, consider himself to be abnormally well-endowed.

Before advising my patient to embark on triple therapy, and especially before committing NHS money, I decided to check her for *H. pylori* antibodies. Her antibody titre should have been off the scale – and she has no detectable antibodies to *H. pylori* at all. Which, as any private specialist will tell you, is not strictly abnormal, but is on the margins of the borders of the lower end of the abnormal range.

Private problems

First came the ENT surgeon who sends his private patients to me to get simultaneous PPI and H_2 blocker treatments in unlicensed doses; second, the private specialist who can't be bothered to order a cheap antibody test when there's a vastly more expensive breath test to be had; and finally the poor sod who had to get a job working in private health care because she doesn't know the difference between being HIV-positive and having full-blown AIDS.

Combine a positive breath test with a neurotic patient and nine days out of ten we'd treat for an easier life

As in, 'Dear Dr Copperfield, your patient consulted today for a health check. She appeared to be unhappy to receive her recent diagnosis of AIDS . . .'

The good doctor mentioned that my patient had AIDS three times in the course of a form letter. The truth is that my patient is HIV-positive. Her counts are good, her loads are tolerable and she's never had anything that even smelt of an AIDS-related condition, let alone the full-blown enchilada.

I wonder what the nice private doctor could have said to upset her?

Give me sick people any day

There's a rumour going round that John Chisholm is on the brink of contacting me to ask my advice on the proposed new contract. I know, because I started it. It's not impossible, is it? 'Tony, me old mucker,' he'd say, 'this contract thing's a right plate of cack and it's doing my head in. Could you have a go?' Stranger things have happened, though I can't think of any.

But, just in case, I'm ready: I have my views on the new contract and it's not just predictable stuff about decapitation fees for heartsinks and free chocolate Hob Nobs for all GPs, though clearly these should be central to any new deal. No, I'm thinking of something more radical. Basically, I don't want to work for the NHS any more. This doesn't mean I've come over all private. It means I want to work purely in the NIS – the National Illness Service.

The argument goes like this. My day can easily be filled by people who are ill. Usually, this illness is not very serious – and, in certain cases, nowhere near as serious as I'd like it to be – but, nonetheless, the punters perceive a real problem and a need for my services, such as a dose of reassurance, a sick note or a poke in the eye for wasting my time.

Vague bell

This all rings a vague bell with why I entered medicine in the first place, which was to treat ill people. Sometimes, I even make ill people feel better, so long as their presenting complaint is ear wax, obviously.

The problem arises with healthy people, or with the 'stabilised ill' in whom we are supposed to prevent complications: the worried well, the smear seekers, the cardiovascular candidates, the diabetics heading for any one of a number of '-pathies', and so on. I'm supposed to keep this little lot healthy too.

Basic grasp

Unfortunately, it cannot be done. Someone with a basic grasp of maths, the back of an envelope and a few minutes to spare recently calculated that simply implementing the cardiovascular NSF would eat up about a quarter of my time, energy and budget. So that means three more NSFs would . . . er . . . oh dear. Besides, I loathe this type of work. It's monotonous, soul-destroying and low-yield: you get lots of unrealistic targets, you make well people feel ill to prevent something which might not have happened anyway, and you get crapped on if it goes wrong.

So sod the NHS, I want to work for the NIS. This is what I trained for, what I enjoy doing and what I can realistically provide. If the politicians still believe in the myth of illness prevention and the patients want a Health Service, then someone else can provide it: I haven't the time and I'm not interested. So split the contract into an 'Illness' Service and a 'Health' Service and have two separate doors into your surgery. In my case, the one marked 'Health' will be permanently locked.

I want to work purely in the NIS – the National Illness Service

And, John, if you're still reading – my e-mail address is right here . . .

The joke's on us – and it's not funny

GPs are very naive. Our patients have known this for years. They know that if they turn up in the first couple of weeks of January, we'll ignore the obvious skiing goggle lines on their faces and will write them a note to confirm that they've been in bed for the past seven days with the winter vomiting bug as opposed to the chalet girl.

The problem is that somebody – probably somebody very high up – in the Department of Health has caught on too, and that somebody is turning out to be a practical joker of the very highest calibre.

Cast your mind back to last year's offering via the primary care tsar, that GPs weren't overworked at all, it was just that we didn't know how to arrange our working day.

In fact, as a gesture of solidarity, he was going to carry on doing the occasional clinical session to show us all how it should be done.

Big bowl

No doubt about it, life as a front-line medic was simply a big bowl of cherries.

Who fell for that one?

Remember the follow-up from Lord Hunt? 'Morale among NHS medical staff was no worse than usual' and doctors in particular were famous for whinging any time they didn't get their own way.

The beatings will continue, of course, until morale improves.

This year's knockabout classic was the spoof story that an academic had proven that GPs have enough spare time to pop in and check on little old ladies on an everyday basis. It fooled hundreds on the Costa Geriatrica.

GPs stupid enough to take the suggestion seriously were soon pounding their stubby webbed fingers into calculator keypads, figuring out that, considering they have 2,164 elderly patients on their list, they would have to devote their entire working day to doing nothing more than toddling from house to house, popping out to the shops for Mrs Incopad to collect her fags and a bit of something for the cat, and running the Hoover around the bedroom carpet.

Women can multi-task and GPs are multi-skilled. So, if female GPs can't manage to write a prescription with their right hand, clean a toilet with their left and clean the floor with a Squeegee mop stuck up their arse, then who can?

Malignant joker

The malignant joker theory would also explain the sudden arrival of 700,000 doses of meningitis vaccine with an imminent sell-by date on the doorsteps of family doctors all over the country labelled, 'Surprise Supplies'.

'It's not fair!' GPs cried. 'We didn't order this,' as though they'd received a selection of books from the militant wing of the *Readers Digest*, accompanied by a demand for payment delivered by a big bloke with a tattooed forehead.

The beatings will continue, of course, until morale improves

More worryingly, they felt that they had to do something constructive with it.

Which was exactly what I did. As with all the other junk mail I get every day, I threw it away.

Tx reviews try my patience

When I began my career in general practice, I had an idea it could get pretty crappy. Over the years, I've shed this initial naivety and discovered that it's much crappier than that.

You'd have thought that, by now, with all my experience, I'd have reached some sort of crap plateau. But no, it continues to be an uphill struggle, as I discover, thanks to new forms of learning – new forms of crap to pile upon the old.

The really galling thing is that some of this faeculent matter is doctor-generated – it comprises sacred cows supposed to represent 'quality care'.

This occurred to me the other day during a consultation with an asthmatic. The poor bloke had gone through the rigmarole of phoning up, booking an appointment, taking time off work and sitting in the waiting room with Basildon's most viral simply because our 'quality' repeat prescribing system had recalled him.

For what? A consultation that basically went: 'How's it going?' 'Fine, thanks' – with a peak flow to pad things out. I don't care what NSFs or the Clinical Governance Gestapo say, it is a waste of time.

Low threshold

My objections are as follows. First, most treatment reviews are unnecessary. Why do I need to check a thyroxine regime annually? Can't we rely on the punters to let us know if there's a problem? They already have a risibly low threshold for attending.

Second, patients can usually monitor their own diseases: they have peak flow meters, BP monitors, pharmacy-based cholesterol tests and so on. I'm potentially redundant, and proud of it.

Third, treatment reviews inevitably create work. If you were an asthmatic, you would not go to the trouble of attending just so the GP could rubber-stamp your repeat prescription. Which is why these patients only ever come when they have some other problem – so a therapy update becomes a 'While I'm here,' and Dr Copperfield becomes hacked off.

Overvaluing illness

Fourth, this is a classic case of doctors overvaluing illness. When will we learn that diseases like asthma or hypertension aren't as important to people as we'd like to believe – not when there's shopping to be done, giros to collect, cars to nick, and so on?

It's absurd expecting patients to take time out from their busy schedules so we can pretend we're providing a quality service. We should realign our values with the punters – in other words, care less.

A therapy update becomes a 'While I'm here,' and Dr Copperfield gets hacked off

After all, the only patient who will attend religiously for treatment reviews is the obsessive basket case who brings a year's worth of computer print-outs depicting his twice-daily peak flow readings. These people shouldn't be encouraged to get to the doctor – they should be encouraged to get a life.

And fifth, treatment review consultations are bloody boring. Which is why I shall overlook one to four above and simply delegate this task to a specialist in the arse-achingly tedious. My practice nurse will be thrilled.

Keep referrals for doctors' eyes only

So, from now on we're supposed to write our medical records and referral letters in simple English, so the elderly and those whose cerebral blood flow is markedly restricted can understand them.

Sorry to spoil the party here, but quite honestly, I don't want any of my patients to have access to their referral letters, or the rest of their notes either.

Ever since the Access to Medical Records Act came into force, I've been plagued by requests from imbeciles to decipher and interpret the abbreviations within their files.

Thankfully, all I have to do is ask them which part of 'access' they found hard to understand. They can borrow, read or copy their notes, even publish them on their Internet homepage, but they've paid their ten quid for access, and that's all they're going to get.

Besides, if granny is going to peruse her medical history then all of her referral letters, and especially those to her ophthalmologist, will need to be typed double-spaced in Arial Bold 48pt, and in capitals too.

Simple English

Translate into simple English this opening sentence from one of my recent referrals to the gynaecology department: 'Dear Slasher, I think you've seen this oligo-synaptic freak of nature in your private rooms, but I can't be sure as you described her as "charming". "Special", as in "needs", would be nearer the mark.'

Or this missive to paediatrics: 'Dear Marion, as soon as I clapped eyes on this web-necked ankle-nibbler, my syndrome detector went off. She was delivered by Bob the Butcher last December but this is one of the rare occasions when I don't think it's fair to blame him for the WLK [weird-looking kid] that resulted.'

Things would be even worse if letters to and from geriatricians were made public. First, they'd have to remove the motto, 'Psychogeriatrics means never having to say you're sorry', from the letterhead and, even worse, they'd find out what 'GOMER', 'LOLINAD' and 'CUBA' really meant.

My trainer (yes, I had one) had two all-purpose referral letters. Letter one ran along the lines of: 'This patient has [a symptom or sign]. Please assess and act appropriately.' The other stated: 'There's sod-all wrong with this patient, but failure to refer him for a pointless second opinion might leave me in breach of my Terms of Service.'

Quite honestly, I don't want patients to have access to referral letters

Readers' wives

One of my letters to obs and gynae, confessing enviously that I wished I could surgically remove all the patient's organs referrable to my specialty, give her an 'I survived surgery at The General' T-shirt and discharge her from follow-up, resulted in a threat to expose me in a learned journal, but the best she could do was have a letter published in the Readers' Wives section of *Men Only*. Along with quite a fetching picture, as it happened.

Finally, if you're the consultant who received my shortest ever referral letter, 'Please look at this kid with a squint. On second thoughts, why not use both eyes?', please take it down from the department's toilet wall forthwith. I know you've had it framed.

Now it's no more Dr Nice-guy

Some of you, I know, believe my rantings are just an exorcism of my darkest thoughts and that, deep down, I'm really Dr Nicey. So I've decided to confess all. I'm not seeking absolution, you understand. I just think it's best that you know what kind of columnist you're dealing with.

First confession: I have an unpleasant Pavlovian set of reflexes to certain key phrases beloved by patients. For example, the fat punter who resorts to: 'I don't eat a thing' inevitably spends the rest of the consultation with a flashing neon sign above his head that reads: 'I'm a lying lard-arse.'

Patients whose opening gambit is: 'I don't know where to start' think my expression is inviting further explanation, whereas it's actually inviting them to stop right there while I take urgent sick leave.

And for those who say: 'I just want a letter,' the unspoken dialogue is: 'Sure, here's a P. Follow that with I, S, S, O, F and F and you might get the message.'

Boring afternoon

This lack of professionalism is not restricted to my thoughts. At times, for fun, I like to talk bollocks, and with great conviction. It is untrue that breathing helium helps asthma, most harmful foods 'begin with T' and antibiotics sometimes make your penis shrink, but I have claimed all these things – to brighten up a boring afternoon, terminate a dull dietary discussion and avoid an inappropriate prescription, respectively.

It gets worse. Sometimes, my attention span is so poor that, once I've taken the history, pretended to examine the patient and drifted into a reverie about future holidays, I've completely forgotten what the presenting symptom is and have to make a wild guess at a plausible diagnosis. Hence consultations ending with the patient saying, slowly: 'So you mean, doctor, that my painful, swollen foot which came on after I was run over by a tractor is actually caused by a virus?' while I nod earnestly.

Sin quotient

Pressure of work really cranks up the sin quotient. If I'm busy and it doesn't suit me for a patient to be hypertensive, I'll knock 20mmHg off his BP reading. If the surgery is heaving, I'll hear that single crepitation to justify an expedient antibiotic. And if I've already sent three in to the medics, then that crushing central chest pain will inevitably sound like oesophagitis.

If I'm less busy, the mischief is pure self indulgence. It's great, for example, examining backs or posterior lung fields because this offers the opportunity to express, via obscene hand signals, what you really think of the patient – though don't try this near any mirrors.

But these sins are nothing compared to the heinous act I committed today. A patient registered blind through severe diabetic retinopathy attended with his guide dog. I like the patient and I like the dog, but I was bubbling borborygmically with last night's curry.

I can't be the first person to have blamed flatulence on a handy animal but, as a doctor, I should be ashamed. It worked well, though.

If I'm busy and it doesn't suit me for a patient to be hypertensive, I'll knock 20mmHg off

Tricks to make mad medical life tolerable

In the 'non-medical interests' section of a previous edition of my CV you'll find my hobbies listed as: 'Join-the-dot puzzles, colouring-in and watching *Teletubbies*'.

You might be relieved to learn this was a spoof résumé designed to ensure I didn't make the shortlist for a job I was being cajoled into applying for and which I would have hated.

Despite a talented field of candidates, I was offered the post, which proves that interviewing panels never actually read the six-page application forms they insist you complete in triplicate.

Despite my published predilection for puzzles aimed at the brain-dead, I don't do mindless things terribly well. If anything, I tend to rebel.

Detailed account

When an insurance company writes to me to ask for a medical report about a patient I am treating for 'Lumbar', I provide a comprehensive and detailed account of the number of consultations we have had about 'Lumbar' (none), the possible complications thereof (none), the currently available treatment options (none), and the prognosis (insufficient data at this time).

So long as they pony up with the forty quid I invoice them for, I might even compose a further report about my patient's sciatica – for another fee, naturally.

Regrettably, there's no such recourse within the NHS. I received a phone message this morning from the occupational therapy department about a patient with a diabetic neuropathy. He swears blind he can't cope at home because of the pain and numbness in his feet and I think he's taking the piss.

I thought I'd send in an OT as a sort of unbiased referee. Can he cope with the varied activities of life, or is he really moribund and bedridden six days out of seven? I know he's fine on Tuesdays because he's always in my waiting room.

Resubmission request

The OT department's message read: 'We cannot accept the referral, please send it again.' Not: 'We will not accept this referral, bugger off' or: 'We cannot accept this referral, send it to another agency', either of which might have been apposite responses.

I know he's fine on Tuesdays because he's always in my waiting room

I love rewriting lost prescriptions. Every line is painstakingly reproduced. Luckily, after signing 70 repeat prescriptions, my inimitable handwriting is totally illegible.

I don't often get asked to perform the task again, and if I am, I've discovered a great trick. Offer to rewrite as many prescriptions as the enemy can throw at you and offer to fax them over to save time. Then write them all with a green ballpoint pen. It'll render them absolutely bloody invisible.

187

Now for something serious

I realise the purpose of this column is to poke patients in the eye, extract urine from the great and good, or simply tickle ribs.

But I do reserve the right to shed my ophthalmic, urological and intercostal role at times and get serious. So, this week, I want to highlight something that isn't at all amusing and that threatens Medical Civilisation As We Know It.

To illustrate: there was recently an article in the *BMJ* that raised some interesting questions about the prostate-specific antigen test. My view is irrelevant, but I'll tell you anyway – I agree with the author's spin that the brakes should be applied to the PSA juggernaut and PSA is really 'persistent stress and anxiety'.

A polarised view, but not, you'd have thought, particularly inflammatory. Wrong. The 'e-response' was huge.

So far, so good – we all love a heated debate. But what was remarkable was not the e-correspondence count, which was impressive, but the content, which wasn't.

Scary group

Because, among the usual academic huffing and puffing, was a scary group of communications from patients and support groups. Their gist may be summarised: I am/know someone who had a raised PSA, it was treated therefore a life has been saved, so to discourage PSA testing is to wish me/my acquaintance dead; you are ignorant/ irresponsible/murderers.

Such polemic is not peculiar to prostates – similar reactions have been provoked by daring to voice scepticism about other sacred cows, such as mammography.

Doctors who discuss chronic fatigue syndrome risk astonishingly venomous flak if their views upset those who monitor the media for the juxtaposition of the letters 'M' and 'E'. And some groups in the US have vitriolically denounced child psychiatrists for 'poisoning' their hyperactive children with drugs such as Ritalin.

Much of this reflex response arises from the punters and their support groups, neither of which are renowned for logic, so maybe we should ignore them.

Aggressive backlash

And fanaticism is nothing new – ask US abortion clinics. But something really unpleasant is snowballing, because doctors who dare to challenge – even in an informed way – risk an increasingly aggressive backlash.

Why? Perhaps the members of our stressed societies have a lower threshold for writer's rage; maybe the information age overloads them with opportunities for venting spleen; perhaps the Internet offers them the chance to fan the flames of extremism.

Doctors who dare to challenge – even in an informed way – risk a backlash

Whatever, the answer must be to put chlorpromazine in the tap water. Failing that, our professional journals should exert some editorial control rather than take the line that all controversy is good.

Someone needs to take this problem seriously, otherwise many of us will be too scared to voice any opinions, and the medical world will be a stagnant place.

It's medical terrorism – and it's not funny.

Straight to the point on MMR

One of these days I know that I'll run out of tales from the dark side of general practice and be put out to stud, or more likely to pasture, in favour of a younger, leaner, meaner and hungrier columnist. In fact, I met my perfect successor the other evening.

He has already triumphed admirably over some seemingly insurmountable social obstacles. He is a mathematician and, even worse, he is French.

He joined in the conversation about the great British public being incapable of understanding the concept of relative risk, in particular about the pros and cons of vaccination. As he specialises in the statistical study of risk, he felt compelled to express an opinion.

I was halfway through a pretzel, and choked in a manner that George Dubya woulda been prouda. 'Sometimes zer people just 'ave to accept zat zer docteurs are right and do az zey are told,' he intoned. This man is a God. Never mind arseing about like me, writing humour columns for the trade press, he should have his own prime-time TV slot.

Endless loop

A few bottles of dry Riesling later, I was locked in one of those endless loops of cross talk that middle-class parents with protruding front teeth get you into.

'Why do all children have to have MMR?' 'Because the benefits to the population outweigh the risk of harm suffered by any particular individual.' 'But what if it's my child who suffers?' Read ad infinitum.

I read in a poem at school that your Mum and Dad screw you up, and I'm always amazed by the resourceful way in which some parents, despite society's best efforts to contain them, come up with new ways to damage their children. Darwinian evolution in action.

Whether we follow the working class moron's 'vaccines are dangerous so my kid ain't getting none' philosophy or the upper-class moron's 'all those vaccines at once? I'll have Jessica done privately' pathway, experience in Ireland and Japan respectively has shown that either course of action results in a rise in what journalists call 'the count'.

Which is probably just what we need. A bit of honest to goodness shroud waving. Over the four-year period after they withdrew their home-cooked MMR vaccine, the Japanese lost 72 children to complications of measles. We lost none. Even the unvaccinated spawn of the unwashed pond life survived, thanks to herd immunity.

So let's see stories in the tabloids about toddlers in body bags cluttering up hospital chapels waiting for a parking space in the mortuary. If a few of them go through the local laundry's 'fast coloureds heavy soil' cycle in the meantime, so much the better.

'Sometimes zer people just 'ave to accept zat zer docteurs are right and do az zey are told', he intoned'

Compared to a standard hospital postmortem examination, half an hour in a tumble dryer really doesn't amount to much, and we need the press coverage.

Ensuing stampede

We all know that more children will probably be injured in the ensuing stampede to get vaccinated than would ever have suffered as a result of the original immunisation programme, but, hey, we don't make the rules, we leave that to the parents – because, if anyone knows what's best for their children, they do. I read it in the papers.

Moving the patient mountain

The penny dropped as I put the phone down on my fifth visit request and looked up at my twelfth 'urgent' of that morning. At the root of all our woes, it occurred to me, is not a lack of money, or inadequate facilities or a shortage of health care professionals. The real cause of our malaise is obvious – it's patients. There are simply too many of the buggers. And, having identified the disease, the cure is obvious – to reduce our workload, we just have to reduce patients.

The trick, I think, is to be radical and proactive. I have a few thoughts on moving the patient mountain which I'd like to share with you. Feel free to send in your own – I shall bundle them all together under the mission statement 'Fewer Patients, More NHS' and send them to that nice Mr Milburn, as he encourages innovation in the health service.

For starters, we should plan ahead for next year's flu season. All we need to do is switch the flu vaccine for something more homoeopathic, such as sterile water, and arrange for some tactical sneezing in the local home for the nearly dead.

MAFF-style cull

Or simply have a MAFF-style cull of the sniffly and all their household contacts, which would have the added benefit of the punters hastily relabelling their colds as 'just colds' rather than 'terrible flu'.

The pharmaceutical companies could also help out. Their manufacturing plants are big places, and it must be very easy for a few neurotoxic contaminants to find their way into the production line – sarin rather than statin, for example. By collaborating with the manufacturers of medical equipment to ensure that sphygmo-manometers read 20mmHg too low and that cholesterol meters automatically knock four off the result, we could achieve impressive cerebrovascular patient reductions a few years down the line. And perhaps the maker of the game 'Operation' could be given the franchise for emergency equipment. I'm sure they'd make a fantastic defibrillator, just like the real thing with a nice red light and buzzer to represent the 'shock', but made from cardboard.

Day out

We shouldn't neglect the elderly, either. Secondary care has done its bit, by putting hospital meals just out of reach, over-polishing floors and making beds that little bit too high. I'd suggest a Government-funded day out to Margate for pensioners who've waited more than six months for their operations. All it needs is a driver with sleep apnoea or a strategically placed patch of oil. Carnage, maybe, but an instant improvement in waiting times for hips and cataracts.

Eradicate long waiting times by eradicating patients

Which leaves us with the delays for outpatient appointments. The solution here is a policy of 'clinic cleansing', in which the health service combines with the armed forces to form the NHSAS. Eradicate long waiting times by eradicating patients – they can run, but they can't hide. And in the orthopaedics clinic, they can't even run.

Then, of course, we start napalm bombing.

Can psychometric tests weed out the psychos?

The media believe that doctors are a bunch of psychologically flawed, drug-abusing drunks who couldn't give a toss if their patients live or die.

I don't know if you took part in that particular survey; I know I did.

Before long you might not have a choice. If the National Clinical Assessment Authority has its way, 'underperforming' doctors referred by their primary care trust will soon be subjected to a barrage of psychometric tests.

So go on, tell me about your childhood. Only joking, I really haven't got the time.

When I was making my way up the greasy pole, I decided that the most effective personality type to adopt would be the sociopath – superficially charming, smarter than most and underneath it all, a bit of a bastard.

But psychiatry has moved on since the days of Eysenck, the anal stamp, and neuroticism.

Screening tests

In the interests of journalism, then, I subjected myself to a selection of self-assessment questionnaires.

Although the NCAA plans to delve only into our personalities, I thought I would break myself in gently with a few screening tests for common psychiatric conditions.

The affective disorder screen took about two minutes to inform me that: 'Your answers reflect the presence of depressive symptoms. It is advised to seek a psychiatric consultation.'

This diagnosis was based on the answers to questions like 'Do you ever feel helpless or that things are slipping out of control?'

Name me a doctor who works in the NHS who doesn't feel that way and I'll buy you a pint.

Moving on to and beyond the anxiety triage: 'Do you have a fear of specific objects, such as knives?' Yes, I bloody well do. Most of the Brentwood Massive are carrying blades.

'Your answers reflect the presence of an anxiety disorder. It is advised to seek a psychiatric consultation.'

I faced up to the New York University School of Medicine Online Screening Test For Personality Disorders. You may as well have a go, too —think of it as a practice run for the real thing.

Shipman Squad

One day the Shipman Squad will break down your door because you referred a heartsink to neurology outpatients solely to get him onto a 15-month waiting list and to give you a 'get out of consultation free' card to cover the next 60 Tuesday afternoon regular-as-clockwork whinges about his funny turns.

Question one: 'Do you suspect that others are exploiting, harming or deceiving you?'

What do they mean 'suspect'? It's bleeding obvious.

Next: 'Are you such a perfectionist that it interferes with your work?'

I also share psychological space with Idi Amin, Stalin and Saddam

Not any more. If I can get to the end of the laughably titled 'emergency clinic' without intentionally harming somebody, then I consider that a result.

According to the PTypes Temperament Test it turns out that I'm a 'rationalist', driven by the need for power and knowledge, but 'hedonist' ran a close second.

This puts me into the frame with John Lennon, Martin Luther King and Albert Einstein. But I also share psychological space with Idi Amin, Stalin and Saddam Hussein.

Any one of the four rational sub-personalities: leader, scientist, inventor or architect, could cross the line to become sadistic, schizotypal, compensatory, narcissistic or schizoid, respectively. I noticed there wasn't a personality type labelled 'doctor'.

Tony Copperfield, Twenty-first Century Schizoid Man. Don't push me.

Sources

- http://www.med.nyu.edu/ Psych/screens/pds.html l
- http://www.geocities.com/ ptypes/temperament_test.html

Stress culture is out of control

I love Jeremy Clarkson, and this is why. In his *Sunday Times* column a few weeks ago, he berated the current compensation culture, commenting that: 'You can sue pretty well anyone for pretty well anything and be assured of a bumper pay day.'

Regular readers will know that my own column is no stranger to criticisms of the legal profession (I believe the specific word I used in a dissection of their chief characteristics was 'twats') and that I have diligently reported instances of ridiculous compensationitis – see 'Copperfield and the female patient who suffered intractable headaches after a tin of rhubarb fell on her head'.

To this should be added the latest absurdity: hot on the heels of the DVT/Pill claim, there are now women coming over all litigious because their doctors gave them so much information that it put them off taking the Pill. You've guessed it – they fell pregnant, so it's the doctor's fault.

It used to be said that we walk a medico-legal tightrope, and it's true, except that now there's not even a tightrope. We're just plunging headlong into oblivion.

Prime catalyst

But I digress. I love Jeremy Clarkson not only because he's been drawing attention to this crap, but because he has cleverly nailed one of the prime catalysts behind the national legal lottery – us. He alleges doctors inadvertently encourage pathetic claims. And he's right. His point is doctors are too fast on the trigger with the label 'stress'. IBS? Stress. Palpitations? Stress. Itchy nipples? Stress. You see a pattern developing? So does he, claiming each time he attends his GP, whether for insomnia, lice or suspected Ebola virus, he's been told it's all down to stress.

This, he suggests, is rubbish, because, 'We were designed to cope with being eaten by a lion'. This explanation doesn't actually reinforce his argument – it would be illogical to be able to withstand the psychological effects of being eaten by a lion, since, after a standard mauling, the physical sequelae, with attendant need for surgery or cremation, would surely override the need for a cuppa and a warm cardy.

Hard cash

But I do take his point – and his conclusion, which is that doctors must stop blaming symptoms on stress, because this simply encourages the punters to take the source of their particular 'stress' to court to convert it into hard cash.

Guilty as charged. I suspect I use stress as my diagnostic catch-all because the patients so readily agree to it. And the previous dustbin diagnosis – 'It's a virus' – has become such a cliché that it's hard to sound convincing and unembarrassed even when it *is* a virus.

The previous dustbin diagnosis – it's a virus – is such a cliché

Perhaps, as the great Mr Clarkson suggests, we should simply be blunt with our patients and point out that their psychosomatic ailments are caused by them being pathetic, spineless morons. Unfortunately, I suspect the psychological trauma of such difficult consultations might bring me out in stress-related hives. So maybe I'll try the 'I think you've been eaten by a lion' line instead. I live in hope.

The fine art of telling them to sod off

There's a TV advertisement that shows an employee of Multinational Energy Corp plc getting out of the bath to answer her phone. It's a wrong number but, rather than doing what any one of us would do, she puts her clothes on and sets off down the road, cordless phone in hand, to the address the caller wanted and knocks on the door.

'Hello,' she says to the bloke who answers, 'call for you'.

I'm not sure if this is supposed to be funny. The problem is my reception staff are starting to behave the same way.

Some of my patients aren't prepared to swallow the standard corporate line about how we handle incoming calls. In particular, they have problems with phone access to the results of their pointless get-the-heartsink-out-of-the-room blood tests and X-rays.

Predictably normal

To provide a better service, as they say, our results line is only available from 11.30am until 3.30pm. This means that patients ringing in with chest pain have at least a fighting chance of getting through and into morning surgery, and that I don't have to start my working day ploughing through a bunch of predictably normal polyinvestograms ordered by over-eager registrars.

It also means that the reception staff can spend time opening the post and throwing away anything on PCT-headed note paper rather than tracking down the result of Mrs Mooncalf's urgent faecal strontium assay.

In reality, the system crashes every morning. I admit I only get to hear one side of the conversation, but the daily mantra goes something like this.

'Hello, my name is Sandra. How can I help you?'

'The result of your test will be available after 11.30, when Dr Copperfield has had time to check it for you. If you ring the "results" number in the practice leaflet around quarter to 12, then. OK?'

'About quarter to 12.'

'It's in the practice leaflet.'

'It's 456227.' '4-5-6-2-2-7.' 'Seven.' 'Yes, quarter to 12.'

'Anytime after 11.30, really, but before 3.30.' 'Three-thirty.' 'In the afternoon, yes.' 'And for X-rays.' 'Yes.' 'No.' 'It's a new system. It saves time.'

'The hospital?' 'I don't think so.' 'The number? Aren't they in the phone book?' 'Not offhand, no.' 'Did they? When?' 'Was that the woman who took the blood?' 'She always says that.' 'I don't think so, but I'll ask. Hang on.'

Essential business

Sandra then asks the practice manager, who is employed on essential biscuit-ordering business, whether she knows the direct-line number for the pathology lab and would it be OK to give it out to a patient.

Some patients aren't prepared to swallow the standard line

I know I'm being unfair. Closing telephone conversations is an art. When I do co-op shifts and have that thing with the three-year-old with earache from the pond-life family who want a visit because the car has a flat tyre, I just say: 'Try these numbers. I'm sure they'll be able to sort something out.'

This teaches the vermin three useful things: first, that I'm smarter than they are; second, that I'm not in the mood to be pissed around; and third, the phone numbers of Kwik Fit and their local minicab office.

Eyes wide open in the new NHS

Spooky. Only a few weeks ago I suggested that the new contract should be split into an Illness Service and a Health Service. So slap my face with a wet kipper, because that's exactly the sort of contract the Great and Good have come up with – if you read 'clinical services' as 'illness' and 'quality' as 'health' – and use your imagination a bit.

So if my articles really do mould the future, I'm looking forward to welcoming Nicole Kidman as our new practice nurse – an event which should certainly provide me with a column.

Meanwhile, back in the prosaic world of the contract, I do believe I've spotted a problem. The new quality system promises to pay us megabucks for jumping through a few number-crunching hoops, defined by the national service frameworks. And the NSFs, as we know, will bust the NHS budget if implemented.

Financial inducements

So, let's think . . . we're going to receive huge financial inducements to create an unaffordable clinical environment. Hmmm . . . well, I've often felt like putting a bomb under the NHS, so I might as well get a reward for lighting the fuse.

But I'm forgetting – Gordon Brown has just promised to pour billions into the health service. So long as he knows those billions will be frittered away getting the nation's collective cholesterol below 5mmol/L, then fine.

I imagine, though, the punters might expect a little more for their money than the promise that they'll die of something other than a heart attack or stroke ten years down the line – but what do I know, I'm just a sodding GP?

And this sodding GP will probably shun the quality stuff altogether. After all, suddenly providing a broadsheet service for my tabloid patients will serve only to confuse them.

Instead, I have a cunning plan – I'm going to make up my earnings entirely from my global sum for 'essential and additional clinical services'. That and the obvious 'wisdom payment'.

Brief interventions

No, I'm not expecting the capitation formula to include special uplifts for patient fetor or for inability to articulate symptoms beyond a farmyard grunt. I'm simply going to need a list size of around 50,000. No problem, I'm into brief interventions.

In fact, I reckon I could take on the whole country's list while the rest of you fanny around trying to get 'quality BPs' of below 150/90 (tip: make them up).

If my articles really mould the future, I look forward to welcoming Nicole Kidman as my new practice nurse

All I'd need is a sort of travelling Copperfield Consulting Roadshow to do the odd surgery in various locations – a bit like the mammography service, but treating ill people, rather than pointlessly squashing breasts.

Some advanced telephone consulting would probably come in handy, too. The vast majority of patient interactions end with an antibiotic, a suggestion they go straight to hospital to see a proper doctor, or an ear syringing. I don't need to be in the same room to sort this out – I just need a phone and a three-sided coin. And the rest, Nicole can deal with.

Kiwis pay a price for charging patients

You're entitled to disregard entirely what I have to say, as this week's column is penned under the combined influence of significant sleep deprivation and a number of units of Bollinger. For I find myself in business class, returning from Auckland.

I won't trouble you with the whys and wherefores. Suffice it to say that this significant jolly means either that the publisher has finally realised the true worth of the Copperfield column, or that he was so fed up with me that he wanted me to bugger off for a bit. I'll let you choose the most plausible explanation.

Whatever, it has been utterly fascinating to take a peek at general practice New Zealand-style. And the really excellent news is that Kiwi GPs are just as burnt out, change-fatigued and pissed off as we are.

It's quite a comfort to know that while we are sleeping, half a world away dissatisfied GPs are treating disgruntled patients and, that when we wake up, it's simply our turn.

Extra irritant

The sources of GP malaise Down Under are many and varied, but pretty much parallel ours. They do have one extra significant irritant, though – the fact that patients pay for their primary care consultations.

Patient charges – ring a bell? Because when the going gets tough, such as any Monday morning at 9.01am, the tough, myself included, get going on the idea of charging patients for consultations.

What an attractive prospect – putting the brake on demand by busting their fag, pub and pizza budget. But if this really is the way we're heading, then, thanks to New Zealand, I've seen the future and the future stinks.

First, consider the associated bureaucracy. Imagine a neat stack of A4 sheets reaching the ceiling. Now imagine putting this stack in a wind tunnel. Finally, imagine retrieving and reordering the stack, while wearing woolly gloves. That's what the paperwork is like.

Second, charging for consultations creates a perverse incentive totally at odds with our current philosophy.

Better things

I've spent years trying to persuade Basildon's most feckless and feeble that I have better things to do than scrutinise their sore uvulas or repeatedly check their blood pressures. Yet the Kiwis are positively encouraging these interactions – because patients mean cash.

But worst of all, it gives patients another stick to beat us over the head with.

We're already berated with gripes that it's impossible to get an appointment, a bugger to find a parking space, a pain sitting in the waiting room, and so on.

The excellent news is that Kiwi GPs are just as pissed off as we are

Add to that: 'It's a bloody waste of my hard-earned cash because you never sort me out', then you have Heartsinks With Attitude and a powerful incentive to prescribe or investigate unnecessarily just to give value for money.

Yikes, and no thanks.

Don't think I've gone completely off the idea of patient charges, though. I'm still in favour of those involving electrodes, genitals and a few thousand volts. Or maybe it's just the champagne speaking . . .

Common sense? Barely a shred of it

Whenever the deadline for this column is looming and my 'ideas pending' tray is devoid of anything publishable, I have come to rely on Mr, Mrs, Ms or Master Phuquit making one of their regular appearances in my hilariously named 'emergency clinic'.

I am no soothsayer, but predict here and now that Mrs P will spend tomorrow lunchtime composing a letter of complaint to my practice manager.

Baby P (normal vaginal delivery at term, fully vaccinated, bottle-fed, 26 weeks old, fit as a butcher's dog) already has four repeat prescriptions set up by gullible assistants and registrars to treat potentially fatal nose snuffles, dry skin and constipation.

Baby P didn't take a dump for 48 hours until this morning, when she did. As Mrs P had already asked to be squeezed in this morning, she thought she'd turn up anyway. Especially —and this is the important bit – as Baby P had sneezed just after her mother had made the phone call. Mr P said that was important and that the doctor had to listen to the baby's chest.

Quick examination

You can guess the rest. Dr C said it wasn't, and he didn't. Dr C did view the child completely undressed, and during a quick abdominal examination to exclude anything worth delaying his coffee break for, was able to discern that Baby P showed no sign of any serious illness. At all. Of any kind. Whatsoever.

You know the stuff – good colour, well hydrated, active and chirpy, no shortness of breath, no signs of difficulty in breathing, no fever, nothing.

Except that Baby P sneezed during the examination.

I won't go into the sordid details about the rest of the interaction. Mrs P wanted her baby's chest listened to, Dr C wanted his logical approach to the management of minor illness listened to. Mrs P wanted more drugs. Baby P didn't need them. Mrs P didn't want to learn what to look out for in terms of early presentations of serious illness. Dr C couldn't be arsed to keep a waiting room full of patients kicking their heels for any longer.

Downward turn

When she brought religion into the conversation, I knew that things were going to take a downward turn. She has the Almighty on her side.

God will provide. I prophesy that baby P will sneeze again before the end of the evening, Mr P will call the deputising service, He will provide a deputy doc who will listen to baby's chest and leave a sachet of amoxycillin with a note suggesting a review the next morning in my 'emergency clinic'.

Baby P showed no sign of any serious illness. At all. Of any kind

God will work a miracle to ensure that deputy doc will mistake perfectly innocent transmitted sounds from a snot-encrusted nose for the cardinal signs of an impending pneumonia. Dr C will suggest X-raying baby's chest to see whether there is a focal infection or not (there never is). Mrs P will go apeshit, rush home and take out the green Biro and lined notepaper.

Dr C will file the letter in the special filing cabinet in the corner – the one that goes 'whirrrrr . . .' as it sucks the paper in.

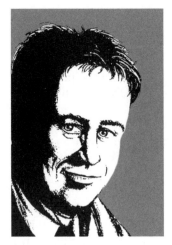

COPPERFIELD CALLING

. . . *Selfridges*

Hello, Selfridges.

Hello. Could you put me through to whoever I need to speak to about Christmas jobs please?

Putting you through. (Pause). Hello, human resources.

I wonder if you could help me. My name's Dr Copperfield, I'm a GP in Essex. I'm a bit fed up and I'm thinking of jacking in the general practice for something more interesting. I wondered if you had any work going over Christmas?

Well, just at the moment, we're –

For example, I'm quite keen on the idea of being the store Santa Claus.

Oh, I see . . .

Yes, obviously, being a GP, I'm quite used to dealing with people, even stroppy ones. I wondered if there are any opportunities at present?

Well unfortunately our Christmas grotto has already opened and we have got quite a few Father Christmases already on board. The only thing is if you write in to us and then we could keep you on hold.

I thought that being a GP might make me a particularly attractive proposition. Do you get many enquiries from doctors wanting to be Santa?

No, not really.

You see, I've done paediatrics, so I'm terribly good with kids. I'd sit them on my knee and everything. I see them every day as a GP, at least for up to seven and a half minutes at a time. I've never frightened one yet.

No, I'm sorry, that really doesn't help.

Anyway, what's the rate of pay for Santa these days?

Two hundred and twenty pounds a week.

Blimey, that's not much. Maybe I'll do a locum instead. What do they do for the rest of the year? Do they get holiday pay?

Er no . . . they're mostly out of work actors.

So you couldn't envisage me having a dual role – you know, being Santa but also being available for any medical emergencies in the store. If there was a cardiac arrest or something I could just whip off the beard and –

Well to be honest, we do have our own occupational health doctors and nurses here anyway, but with regards to Father Christmases, I have actually filled them all.

It's a pity really. You could have had some system for calling me if there were any emergencies, like Rudolph's red nose flashing or something. And my elves could have brought the crash trolley.

Unfortunately I don't think we could do that.

Thanks for your help all the same.

You're welcome.

Oh, and Happy Christmas. Ho ho ho.

Ha, yes. Happy Christmas.

Standing up for men's sexual health

If I ever have the chance to 'do a Paxman' on a health minister, I know exactly what I'll do. I'll prove that politicians are totally incapable of saying the word 'rationing'.

This I'll achieve by getting them to say, in quick succession, words like 'rat', 'rational' and 'ratatouille'. Then I'll throw in 'rationing' and watch them splutter and stutter with that strange, specific dysphasia which results from the lobotomy all politicians are presumably obliged to have.

By simply getting the politicians to say 'rationing', we might at least be able to start a sensible debate on the subject. And nowhere is this more pressing than in men's health: specifically, the ludicrous restrictions placed on treatments for erectile dysfunction.

If the Government can ration in an outrageously arbitrary way, then so can I, which is why Southampton supporters and men with mullets on my list are no longer entitled to any form of NHS treatment.

Hot potato

But why revisit the knackered subject of ED treatment rationing? Because it's a hot potato again. Those Who Know say that most ED is caused by vascular insufficiency. So a man saying, 'While I'm here . . .' with hand on doorknob and eyes cast groinwards, is now a spot diagnosis of atherosclerosis.

These punters should be worked up as though they've presented with angina. Which will work them up: 'You're impotent but, hey, it won't be for long, because your heart's probably buggered, too.'

If you accept that (1) ED really is a sign of vascular disease, and either (2) we're GPs on a mission to rescue men from atherosclerotic hell or (3) we're GPs who've had compliance with statin and aspirin prescribing bludgeoned into us with a rolled-up cardiovascular national service framework, then the conclusion is clear. We should be encouraging men with ED to attend.

But isn't this difficult to square with politicians' policy of denying the majority of men sildenafil *et al* on the NHS?

How does the Government get away with it? In the same way it gets away with pouring vast resources into the dodgy and exclusively female activities that are cervical and mammographic screening.

Medical sexism

In the same way that it gets away with providing free contraception for women while men have to cough up for condoms. In the same way that it promotes the concept of catering for women who want to see a female GP while there is never a murmur about a reciprocal arrangement for men. It's sexism in medicine, and it happens because men's health isn't politicised.

Sexism in medicine happens because men's health isn't politicised

Consider how many women receive HRT for dubious indications. Imagine the outcry if HRT were restricted to women who have suffered a premature menopause. And yes, I know all about osteoporosis prevention, but ED treatment helps mend marriages, too – or are fractured female bones valued above fractured relationships?

The restricted provision of ED therapies in the NHS is a blatant example of what I've been saying. Ask any politician, he'll tell you – it's ratatouille.

I'm not here to do hand-holding

There I was, nose to nose with a bloke who wanted me to drop everything and accompany him to the home of a patient who had died unexpectedly the previous night.

He wanted a doctor out so, when he broke the bad news to the oblivious widow, a qualified physician would be on hand to administer succour, prescribe benzodiazepines and to make tea for the grieving.

Several occasions

That is so not what I do – although, according to his story, many of you have helped out in the past, because he's done this on several occasions.

I don't know what you guys spend your days doing if you've got time to ride shotgun with do-gooders, but I should keep it very quiet, if I were you – at least until the new contract negotiations are over. Some of us have to work at practising medicine for a living.

The clue I missed, Conan Doyle fans will have noticed, was that my opponent across the reception top had previous convictions for this offence.

I went into the 'bereavement is not an illness, it's a part of normal human experience, what you need isn't a doctor, it's a priest . . .' routine. There's only one way to top that, and he did. 'I am a priest.' Arse.

210

Falling back on the 'but the woman isn't even my patient, she's registered with the surgery down the road' ploy did little to help. I didn't even mention that, as she wasn't my responsibility, if he persisted with his crazy request I'd be happy to send him a bill for medical services rendered at £155 per hour, including travel.

He had the moral high ground. I had a surgery full of heartsinks demanding to be seen within 20 minutes of their appointment time, in line with current Blairite guidelines, or be given a cogent reason why they were being kept waiting.

Mindless inadequates

As an excuse, 'You're being kept waiting because you're a load of mindless inadequates with no other place to go on a Tuesday morning, otherwise, why would you be here at all?' doesn't have PCT approval yet, but I'm working on it.

I was wishing that I could do what they do in *ER* at times like this, and tell the reception staff to call security, when a bloke in a black outfit and a peaked cap, bearing the legend 'Security' appeared out of nowhere.

I went into the 'bereavement is not an illness, you need a priest not a doctor' routine

It didn't actually matter that he looked about as threatening as Dale Winton and wore the happy-go-lucky smile of a Springer spaniel that had just been shown a card trick. He was on the premises, in uniform and on duty, as a reaction to the news that a local lunatic, recently released from prison, had made death threats against the baby clinic staff.

Planning to assassinate health visitors isn't lunacy, it's just thinking outside the box about NHS cost-effectiveness.

In any case, the priest accepted defeat when he saw the cattle prod.

But hold on, I get death threats on a regular basis, and the PCT doesn't send a liveried jobsworth to protect me. I can't even get so much as a drug company-sponsored flak jacket.

Maybe I should go into paediatrics.

Get me a gun
. . . a nice gun

I look from the little girl to her mother. 'She's got allergic rhinitis,' I explain. 'Like hay fever, except she's allergic to her rabbit, not pollen.'

I turn back to the little girl. 'What's your rabbit's name?'

'Bugs,' she whispers.

'Okay. Well, the good news is we can make your runny nose better.' I lean closer to her. 'But the bad news is you've got to shoot Bugs.'

Patient-centred

Which reminds me: the Department of Health has the barefaced cheek to suggest that we doctors aren't 'nice enough' to our patients. Apparently, newly qualified doctors and nurses are to receive 'lessons in being nice'.

You'll assume I'm making this up, so here's a quote from the story on the BBC news health website to prove it: 'We want all staff in the NHS to be given training with a patient-centred focus.'

Now there's a novel idea. Let's become patient-centred. Let's improve access, involve them in decisions, prolong their consultations, and provide them with a 24-hour helpline to plug the few remaining moments devoid of medical entertainment.

Oddly, these ideas ring a bell – as does the sound of patients throwing tantrums when they don't get their own way because they've been indulged like two-year-olds who firmly believe they're the centre of the universe.

If only I'd realised I suffer violence and abuse as a GP simply because I'm not being nice enough. How could I have been so stupid? All I need to do is compliment the patient on the attractive 'love/hate' tattoos on her knuckles and never again will I hear: 'Fat lot of f***ing use you are,' when I decline an antibiotic.

As I move onto advanced niceness, I shall end each consultation with a hug and maybe, then, they'll stop gobbing on my car.

Empathy slime

I hate to state the bleedin' obvious, but if anyone needs lessons in being nice, it's the punters. I spent most of my VTS enduring earnest talks from hand-wringing twats with cardies for brains teaching me how to be touchy-feely. By the time I saw my first real primary care patient, I was leaving a trail of empathy slime wherever I went.

I learned quickly, though. That first patient was a junkie on the scrounge for anything ending in '-pam'. His opening gambit was: 'Give me a prescription or I'll kick your bastard head in.'

If only he'd had the benefit of the Department's Lessons in Niceness, he might have tried: 'Give me a prescription or I'll kick your bastard head in, please, doctor' – then he might have got somewhere.

Apparently, newly qualified doctors and nurses are to receive lessons in being nice

All this tripe about patient-centredness just softens us up when we should be developing thicker skins. How else are we supposed to cope with escalating complaints, cussedness and emotional incontinence?

Over her wailing, I say, smiling: 'Just kidding. You don't have to shoot your rabbit.'

'No?' She sniffs.

'No,' I reassure her. 'I'll do it for you.'

Zen and the art of patient placation

As a GP, I have good days and bad days. I shuttle between mildly indifferent and frankly uninterested. Now and again I reach the heights of nirvana, attaining, 'can't give a toss' status for a fleeting moment before returning to the physical world and its trials – namely Julia Scrag and her performing troupe of Scragettes, who are currently trashing my partner's consulting room. I'm not having those little bastards barfing into my wastepaper bin again.

Because I never actually do anything, apart from repeat Copperfield's Medical Mantra 'it's only a virus, it's only a virus' at seven-minute intervals, it's difficult for my allocation of poorly-evolved knuckle-draggers to get snotty about the way I do business.

When they complain, I simply open my book of Evidence-Based Medicine and point out that nothing I'm allowed to prescribe would make any difference anyway.

Blissful ignorance

Doctors in cardigans who really care go apeshit about drugs with an NNT of six, blissfully ignoring the fact that the vast majority of the poor bastards they are poisoning with them will get nothing but side-effects.

Like I worry. If Mrs Scrag wants to insist that her tribe will only stop chucking up at one end and leaking at the other if they get their fortnightly ration of antibiotics, then tough – and, after the erythromycin and metronidazole combination kicks in – even runnier stuff for the herd.

She's hardly likely to complain about the rivers of diarrhoea trailing behind her kids if she knows it's being treated proper 'wiv an antibiotic'.

The problem is, I am torn. Patients can now complain successfully that their GP did not persuade them strongly enough to smoke less and have their screening tests.

Anyone who so much as dips into this column must realise that I believe screening to be a steaming pile of pseudo-scientific cack. The only reason I suggest heartsinks have screening tests is the hope that they'll suffer when false positives result in painful further investigation and unnecessary surgical procedures.

Smoking perils

But be warned, unless you spend hours of your life tacking little addenda on to your consultations about the perils of smoking and the joy of slimming clubs, or reminding people to have their smears and cholesterol checks, then your arse is on the line.

You have an overwhelming responsibility for your patients' welfare. Or do you? What about your responsibility to humanity as a whole? Wouldn't the world be a better place if we could shed a few hundred thousand of the hoi polloi? The sort of people who need the warning 'Contains Nuts' on a peanut choccie bar.

There are some messages sentient human beings only need to hear once

There are some messages that sentient human beings only need to hear once. Don't drive without a seat belt, don't eat the yellow snow, that sort of thing.

Those cute'n'cuddly chain-smoking lard-arses spend years of their lives working toward an early demise. Is it really ethical to stand in their way?

A classic case of damage limitation

It's Sunday, it's 3pm, and I'm on duty. I look at the phone, because I know it's going to ring. It rings. 'Hello, Mrs D,' I say, before Mrs D – for it is she – can utter a word.

Oh joy. Mrs D complains of chest pain and dizziness. Again. She's had these symptoms all her life. Her first words as a toddler were: 'I've got chest pain and dizziness,' closely followed by: 'Get the doctor.'

I'm not sure if the unborn can get chest pain and dizziness but, if they can, the foetal Mrs D suffered them and only failed to call because there are no phones *in utero*.

Three o'clock seems to be the only time of day she's on her own so, naturally, she rings us for reassurance. The conversations are stereotyped – 'So it's the same chest pain and dizziness you've always had, Mrs D. Excellent. Same time again tomorrow, then.'

Defending inaction

But the entries in the notes aren't stereotyped. Instead, they show an interesting evolution. Initially, there were screeds hypothesising on cardiac or respiratory causes. As repeated investigations drew a blank, and time – and Mrs D – went on and on, they became more succinct and oriented towards defending inaction.

Hence: 'Nil to suggest a cardiac problem.' But now, we can't even be arsed to do that. So the three latest entries read: 'Usual problem; usual advice'; 'The usual'; and 'Ditto'. The challenge to better this is irresistible so, besides the date, I just put: 'Zzz.'

We've given up trying to make a diagnosis or shake her faith in her symptoms; our strategy is damage limitation. Mrs D needs protecting from hospitals, and hospitals certainly need protecting from her.

And it's a triumph that we've managed to conceal from her the number of NHS Direct, for this would be a marriage made in hell. When she asks, I give her pizza home-delivery numbers instead. Same concept, tastier outcome. And a deep-pan pepperoni is a small price to pay for not paralysing the NHS.

This is what worries me about the great, easy-access, customer-friendly, nurse-led, protocol-driven NHS we're developing. There are plenty of Mrs Ds around, and they can only be effectively handled by people who know their patients, who are prepared to take risks and who can cope with uncertainty. That's us.

Important attribute

Plug these nightmares into an NHS-By-Numbers and the system will implode within days.

The other important attribute we GPs have is a self-preserving fatalism. One day, Mrs D's chest pain and dizziness will be caused by an infarct, and we'll miss it. We must do, because the alternative is to send her to hospital for ECGs and cardiac enzymes every single day.

Her first words as a toddler were: 'I've got chest pain and dizziness'

The lesser evil, which you won't find in any protocol, is to accept we'll foul up sometime. But, hopefully, that'll be when she's old enough for it not to matter. Any time now, in fact.

So if the phone doesn't ring at 3pm tomorrow, I'll miss it, oddly. And I'll think, regarding today's conversation: 'Oops.' But that's all.

When in doubt, leave it to the professionals

The last time I put a house on the market I asked the estate agent to include the wording 'professionally tiled bathroom' in his details. He looked at the less-than-perfect grouting and gave me one of those sideways looks that meant: 'You cannot be serious'. It was tiled by a doctor and a barrister on their weekend off, and you don't get much more professional than that.

So what exactly does it take to be a 'professional'? I ask because everybody, it seems, wants to get in on the act. Nurses are now professionals, refuse collectors are now professionals, homoeopaths are now professionals. It can't be anything to do with the length of time spent training for the job, as apprentices spend seven years learning their chosen trade and seem to be quite content to refer to themselves as 'craftsmen'.

Neither is it anything to do with intellect. Even applicants whose lips moved as they read the advertisements inviting them to 'Join the Professionals' were more than likely to be accepted, with or without GCSEs, and at the end of their training were fully entitled to describe themselves as professional soldiers.

If nurses are allowed to join the elite band, it certainly can't be related to dedication to the job. If it were, could any group of workers whose regulatory body could well be termed 'Ofsick' honestly expect to join the select few?

I think it boils down to a couple of issues. A previous US president had a sign on his desk in the Oval Office that read 'The Buck Stops Here'. When you're entitled to call yourself a pro, if things go wrong then it's in the job description that you take the flak. It will be interesting to see how that pans out when nurses get their hands on prescription pads.

The first time a punter gets poisoned by a toxic drug combination, will the 'professional' nurse who signed the FP10 be there? Or will the doctor who signed off her training for the relevant Patient Group Directive – or whatever they're called these days – find a letter on his doormat on GMC notepaper?

A friend who works for the BBC, and who could easily cost the licence payers a couple of million if she inadvertently libelled a multinational, pays about £300 per annum in malpractice insurance. We pay ten times that or more. I wonder how nurses' indemnity premiums will reflect their new-found status?

When a punter gets poisoned by a toxic drug combination, will the 'professional' nurse who signed the FP10 be there?

Secondly, professionals don't stray outside the boundaries of their expertise. What do those signs that advertise 'Architect Designed Apartments' actually mean? Who else could do the job? I don't expect or want advice about proton pump inhibitors from ENT surgeons or cardiology opinions from dermatologists, however well meant.

Ask anybody. Their butcher may be a fine tradesman, their car mechanic a skilled engineer, their joiner and carpenter a craftsman, but their GP is a professional, because if and when the brown stuff hits the fan, we don't get to duck.

Can't we just knock PDPs on the head?

Er hello? Weren't we all supposed to be appraised this year? Have the Clinical Governance Prefects left me out because I'm obviously beyond redemption? Possibly not, because none of my colleagues have been appraised, either. Nor have they heard of anyone who's heard anything about even the merest whiff of a possibility of being appraised.

In short, it's just not happening. OK, the year of reckoning has only just begun. But you'd have thought there'd at least be the faint rumble of eager appraisers about to appear on the horizon, clipboards in hand and earnest expressions on face. There isn't.

Which is excellent, because I can thumb my nose at those who prissily told me: 'You can't ignore it, it won't go away, you know.' Because I have, and I think it might. Show me all these would-be appraisers. Who's got the time? Who's got the inclination? And who wants to take the flak when a successful appraisee turns out to be 'Shipman: the sequel'?

'Hmm, maybe I fulfilled one educational need too many with that session on proactive terminal care.' No thanks – I have enough trouble justifying my own actions without being tangentially responsible for those of the mad and bad.

But, should they come knocking on my door, I'll be ready. Where's my PDP? Eaten by a patient's guide dog. Or struck by a meteorite. Or whatever.

You see what appraisal will do? We'll end up like junkies thinking of excuses for lost scrips. Alternatively – also like junkies – we'll learn the art of forgery, cobbling together a PDP in the time it takes to remember what it stands for.

Maybe I'll just tell the truth. I haven't got a PDP. I find the whole concept of stating my learning objectives and collecting information patronising and indulgent. I refuse to turn my professional life into a stupid scrapbook for rubber-stamping by some officious prat. There's no time and no need. Anyone who's already doing this isn't a reflective learner, he's an underemployed tosser. I loathe being instructed to reflect on what I do. Anyone with a grain of professionalism and self-respect does this automatically. If I'm the sort of person who needs this pointed out as an 'idea', then I'm the sort of person who wouldn't bother and wouldn't learn from it anyway.

Continue this unrealistic, puerile, time-consuming charade on a five-yearly cycle, and, it seems, you'll be revalidated.

I refuse to turn my professional life into a stupid scrapbook for rubber-stamping by an officious prat. There's no time and no need

Look, I'll do you a deal. I'll take revalidation on the chin; it's just the process I can't bear. Take the pain away – just give me a five-yearly half-hour MCQ to prove I'm up to speed. This would put the 'valid' into revalidation more painlessly than any other scheme. But fat chance, because it seems the wheels may be moving after all. Apparently, there's a reappraisal 'toolkit' in the pipeline. I hope, like other toolkits, it contains a big, heavy spanner. If so, my appraiser would be well advised to wear a helmet.

You can't legislate for wilful stupidity

You probably didn't see it. The British Heart Foundation used an image of a patient with a polythene bag over her head to illustrate the symptoms of heart failure.

Every patient I meet knows exactly what heart failure is, because all their relatives died of it. 'Heart failure is when the heart, yunno, fails, innit? It sort of stops. Like when it's failed. That's why you die.'

There are 800,000 patients with cardiac failure in the UK, and it's fair to assume that they know the symptoms. It was their idea to use the image because it symbolised exactly how they felt fighting for breath.

I distinctly remember seeing a public information film when I was a kid. A cartoon about a bunny rabbit bounding across the meadow but, tragically, during one of his graceful arcs over the buttercups, he managed to dive head-first into a polythene bag, carried along by the breeze.

A few seconds of animated twitching later, it was over. A cotton-tailed corpse lying motionless on the grass. Fade to end title: 'Don't drop litter.'

Not, as I recall, 'Don't drop litter. And don't be stupid enough to put a polythene bag over your head either.' There didn't seem to be a need.

Back to the BHF campaign. End result: several thousand requests for information about heart failure and a rap across the knuckles from the Advertising Standards Authority for using such a potentially dangerous image.

The ASA can try all it likes to protect people from themselves but we GPs do not have that luxury. If we are going to retain even the last vestiges of our sanity working in the remnants of the NHS, then we have got to accept one basic truth: we can't save them all. Some of our patients will die in their sleep because their time has come. Some will die because somebody – on current evidence, a junior hospital doctor from Portsmouth – won't know enough medicine to save them. And a few will die because a bizarre sequence of unconnected and usually unimportant oversights conspire to finish them off – Copperfield's Shit Happens Syndrome. Many, though, will expire as a result of their own stupidity.

Despite scientists' best efforts to perfect the Idiot-Proof World, there are thousands working to perfect The Better Idiot through the genetics of inbreeding.

Some of our patients will die in their sleep because their time has come. Many, though, will expire as a result of their own stupidity

I think I've confessed before to my fondness for those 'How to treat a difficult case of . . .' columns in the medical press. I read one recently along the lines of, 'Sharon, a 23-year-old, 40-a-day Marlboro Light smoker, has read in the tabloids that smokers who eat strawberries don't get cancer. How do you respond?'

Cue GP commentator adamant that the first thing you must do, after you've empathised or sympathised or whatever, is to use all your powers of persuasion and all the time allocated to your coffee break to get her to change her life and quit smoking.

But why bother with all that? A cheery, 'Yes, I read that too,' is all you need.

Telling it like it is – 'You can try it if you like, dog breath, but the only benefit is that you might die before you reproduce' – might cause offence.

It's time to book myself into an old folks home

Over the years, I've suffered many home visit embarrassments. Encouraging a mangy, loitering dog into a patient's house and onto his sickbed, for example, mistakenly thinking the patient was the owner. Being incapable of retracing my route from a patient's bedroom to the front door, so that I wandered around like a retarded rat in a maze. And resuscitating a diabetic in a hypo, armed only with a 2ml syringe – yep, that's 25 mini-squirts of dextrose. But I've recently managed to top these.

The call was from one of our two local nursing homes for a lady who was 'off her legs'. These calls elicit an unpleasant Pavlovian reflex, for the simple reason that they're almost always rubbish.

You know the type of thing. The symptoms of the barely sentient are Chinese-whispered among only slightly more sentient staff, to be presented to the doctor by someone who learned their logic and clarity at the School for Railway Tannoy Announcers – and who knows to end every message with 'straight away please'.

Given the interruption to afternoon surgery, and the likely shambles ahead, I managed to work myself up to a nicely explosive pitch of irritation en route. So I wore a menacing look as I strode purposefully and pompously into the nursing home.

I barked at the nearest member of staff, 'So where's Mrs Grunge, whom I've been called urgently to assess?' My lips curled nicely into a sneer with the word 'urgently' and I spent the next few moments refining my 'I'm an important doctor in a hurry, and you're a bunch of morons' expression.

The staff looked at each other in confusion. One was eventually brave enough to speak. 'I'm sorry Dr Copperfield, I don't know anything about this. And I don't actually know where Mrs Grunge is.'

I snapped. Fourteen years of suppressed, nursing home-induced vitriol erupted. 'Bloody hell!' I roared. 'This really takes the sodding Rich Tea biscuit! You drag me out of surgery for an emergency and you don't even know where the patient is! You should be ashamed of yourselves, sitting around on your fat arses while the rest of us are trying to hold the NHS together. This is a load of . . . of . . .' I scrabbled frantically for an appropriately blistering, expletive-loaded and irrefutable phrase, '. . . of pants,' I said, finally. Because something had rather taken the wind out of my sails.

Matron had arrived and was looking, first quizzically, then amusedly, at the patient's records. Then she very gently broke it to me that I was in the wrong place. I had visited the wrong nursing home.

She led me gently back to the front door in a practised manner she'd used, I could tell, with the dribbly and incontinent. And though I wasn't dribbly, I had, by now, wet myself

She told me this with great compassion as she gently led me back to the front door, in a practised manner she'd used, I could tell, with the dribbly and incontinent. And, though I wasn't dribbly, I had, by now, wet myself.

Later, I reflected on this incident and asked a respected colleague what he thought.

I imagined he'd say I was stressed, overworked, heading for burn-out. He didn't. 'Tony,' he said, 'this simply means you're a pillock.'

It ain't over till the fat lady counts to four

They say if you buy a man a fish you feed him for one night, but if you teach a man to fish you turn him into a bore who buttonholes you in the pub and regales you with tales about the ones that got away.

Of course, this all depends on the bloke in question being able to learn in the first place.

I don't know how many of you prescribe anti-obesity drugs to patients. In my view, not nearly enough of you. Any product that causes those who can consume an entire pig at a single sitting to kak their pants or worse, ought to be promoted as strongly as possible. However, there are rules limiting their use, so to make the lives of our practice staff simpler, I produced an easy-to-use algorithm detailing the pre-treatment requirements, weight and blood pressure checks and milestones for continuing treatment for each drug.

What I had forgotten is that nurses can't do maths. Nursing home staff in particular (but the hypothesis probably extends to nurses in general), cannot count beyond the number four.

No matter how many patients need to be seen in the clinic, a message will invariably arrive that no more than four need to be assessed. When the doctor has seen all the patients listed and makes to leave, the nurse will simply feign surprise and insist that there are many more people to see.

I used to puzzle about this. I even wondered whether they thought that keeping the true number secret was considered to be an act of kindness in nursing circles. The only explanation that holds water, though, is that nurses count using a similar system to the Eskimo: 'One, two, three, four, lots'. They would never dare tell the visiting GP there are 'lots' of patients to deal with, so they settle for the highest number they know – three or four, depending on their level of training.

Anyway, back to the story. Mrs Lard, who had (and probably still has) a BMI pushing 37, was very pleased when I suggested she try one of the NICE-approved cures for overeating.

After she failed – inexplicably – to lose the required tonnage to qualify for one anti-obesity drug, despite a virtually fat-free diet over four weeks, I handed over a month's supply of another before passing her over to our caring and capable nursing staff.

No matter how many patients need to be seen, a message will invariably arrive that no more than four need to be assessed

Four weeks later the Lard file (almost as fat as its subject) was in my pigeon hole. She had managed to gain 4kg (or 'lots', possibly) during her first month on treatment.

Fastened to the record was a note from the nurse: 'Does she have to stop taking the pills?' Helpfully, I returned the notes to her with another copy of 'Copperfield's Easy Algorithm for the Hopelessly Fat' – weight loss targets and all. Next day the file came back, bearing another note, 'Tony, stop being funny, does she have to stop taking the pills or not?'

Time to get real on quality targets

People, I have scary news. Someone out there is talking sense. What's more, he's a specialist. And he might just salvage our profession.

So let's doff our caps to Dr Peter Winocour, consultant physician at the QE2 hospital, Welwyn Garden City. For it was he who provoked in me an extraordinary and unprecedented reaction: I kissed my copy of the *BMJ*. His article on page 1,577, 29 June issue, is worth a foul taste in the mouth. The title says it all: 'Effective diabetes care: a need for realistic targets'.

I can't recall ever having seen the word 'realistic' in any learned journal. And this is precisely what's wrong with research, guidelines, EBM and all the other flim flam that constrains how we work – they're all completely unrealistic. Now, at last, this fact has been acknowledged – in a proper journal, by someone who sounds like he knows what he's talking about.

In case you missed it, Dr Winocour points out that the current targets for glucose, lipid and BP control in diabetics are achievable in only 50 to 70 per cent of patients in research studies. And, as we all know, research patients are from Mars, real punters are from Basildon.

He also states, bravely, that these targets are impractical and involve absurd polypharmacy. When I read this, I confess I began strutting the floor with chest puffed out and fist clenched, screaming 'Yes! Yes!' in a manner usually reserved for England versus Argentina matches ending 1–0 to the Ing-er-lund.

I have but two small regrets. First, that the Copperfield column is not cited as a reference. After all, I have been saying exactly the same thing for the past two years. Remember my insightful piece suggesting that diabetics should be allowed a maximum of four different pills, with any addition requiring a balancing subtraction – start a statin, stop a beta blocker.

And my plea for creative sphygmomanometry in which we knock, say, 20mmHg off each reading. Both caused little impact, unlike Dr Winocour's piece, probably because he has rather more authority.

Second, I feel sceptical about one of his conclusions, which is that the pharmaceutical industry should develop combination tablets to overcome the problem of multiple pill taking. Since he points out that the average diabetic is likely to end up on at least nine different treatments, this combi-tablet would need to be the size of a hockey puck.

These are but minor flaws, though. I would like to propose that Dr Winocour be invited to lead a new and very necessary body, 'The National Institute for Pragmatism' (NIP) through which all guidelines, protocols, NSFs and so on should pass for reality testing. Set this up to NIP all nonsense in the bud and I might decide that I can bear to continue being a GP for a few more years. So Dr Winocour, I salute you. And if I ever develop diabetes, I'm heading straight for Welwyn Garden City.

As we all know, research patients are from Mars, real punters are from Basildon

The bucks go where the buck stops

One of our registrars read this entry in the medical record of one of her patients this morning: 'Spot-the-ball Health visitor can only palpate one testis. I can palpate both. This is why I get the big bucks and she doesn't. TC.'

I have no recollection of the consultation or its documentation, but it's the sort of thing you might reasonably expect to find in the files of any of my patients who have escaped the Thames Gateway towns and ended up registering with you.

All this stuff about nurses being professionals and GPs being replaced with androids working to PCT protocols by the year 2007 got me thinking: why do I get the big bucks?

I don't get enough bucks, obviously, and neither do you, but I get bigger bucks than the health visitors, the nursing staff and anybody else in the primary care network.

Yesterday, it all became clear to me – I get the big bucks because I deserve them.

Percy, a 97-year-old inmate of the twilight zone known as the elderly Mentally Infirm Unit (locked), climbed over the cot sides and fell from his bed in the small hours of Saturday morning, sustaining a shallow five-centimetre laceration to his left forearm. You know the sort of thing – a few layers of epidermis scraped away to form an angry-looking red wound healing by granulation.

The night staff bandaged the correct arm (either by a lucky guess or the flip of a coin) and, to cover their backsides, referred him to the Saturday morning day staff. The day staff took down the dressing, cleaned the wound, stuck some Steristrips across the tissue-paper skin he'd lacerated, re-dressed the wound, and then – to cover their backsides – referred Percy to the senior nurse on duty. She then took down the dressing, inspected the wound and decided to cover her backside by referring Percy to the visiting community nurse on Sunday afternoon.

The district nurse took down the dressing, inspected the wound and – to cover her backside – suggested that Percy be sent to the local A&E department forthwith.

The matron, calculating the staffing and transport costs involved in transferring Percy for a seven-hour wait in A&E at time-and-a-half, covered her backside financially by suggesting that instead of sending him out, he should be assessed by the doctor-on-call service.

The deputising doctor asked the nursing staff to take down the dressing so that he could inspect the wound. Then – to cover his backside – he prescribed a course of anti-biotics for a 'pre-visible cellulitis' and suggested that Percy be reviewed by his own GP at the earliest opportunity.

Our decisions cover the backsides of an entire food chain

His own GP saw him Monday evening and simply said: 'Stop. For Christ's sake, stop. Stop tearing more flesh away every time you take down the dressing. And then get some taller cot sides.'

Percy's fine, by the way, and his wound is healing as quickly as anybody could expect a nonagenarian's forearm to heal.

The reason why you and I get the big bucks is because our decisions cover the backsides of an entire food chain.

Pulling the woollie over doctors' eyes

Some salivate over stamps. Others spot trains. Me? I'm an obsessive collector of daft courses. I don't actually attend any of them. In fact, the thrill of avoidance is part of the fun. The rest is the pleasure I derive from some of the course titles.

A few are simply bizarre. In the past few years, locally, we've had 'Ladder care', a 'Fire awareness day', and a course in 'absence', which I suspect was poorly attended. Some seem plain unnecessary, such as the recent seminar on 'Assertiveness for nurses' – if the nurses I know were any more assertive, they'd have Lennox Lewis hiding behind his mother's legs.

But most of my collection is reserved for courses that are frighteningly touchy-feely cardie magnets. Collecting them gives me a guilty exhilaration, a little like having a secret stash of pornography: naughty, rather alien, and a place I Know I Dare Not Go, as it might pervert me forever.

Until recently, my favourites were a course entitled 'Complaints are useful' – yeah, right – and another under the auspices of 'The Alchemy Foundation of Holistic Science', called (I kid you not) 'The bridge of light diploma in metaphysics'. Which I think is self-explanatory.

I say until recently, because someone who is aware of my strange course fetish kindly sent me the programme for WONCA's UK conference. I appreciate that WONCA is a pretty soft target, not least because imaginative manipulation of one of its vowels perhaps tells you all you need to know about the organisation.

And I realise they have to provide a broad and varied programme. But, frankly, I'm ashamed of a profession that can promote talks such as, 'Approaching the strong points of our patients', 'The wounded GP', 'Dealing with crying patients' (I find Kleenex and the door work well) and 'Imagination and empathy in the consultation'. Or which asks you, in a keynote talk, to 'celebrate a unique encounter with the undiagnosed human being'. Wishful thinking where I work – as some of my patients are more likely to provide unique encounters with undiagnosed protozoa.

The only title that set my pulse racing was the enigmatic: 'The role of flying nurses in preventive work'. Now there's an idea: fill up a Hercules with a dozen nurses and drop them from a great height on smoking punters. And perhaps this explains 'The wounded GP' – struck by a low-flying nurse?

The point is that, over the past ten years or so, medical education has become increasingly earnest, hand-wringing and fluffy to the point that it has no real substance. Where are the real life, common-sense, practical sessions that would improve my working day? Who is catering for GPs who want a session on 'The no-touch consultation'? Or a course on 'How to refuse antibiotics in ten different languages'? Or a seminar on 'Fumigating your room after a visit from Mrs Lard: air freshener, open windows or a masking burst of flatulence?' No one. Still, that's my learning needs sorted for this year.

Most of my collection is reserved for courses that are frighteningly touchy-feely cardie magnets

It's a bum job – but someone has to do it

I once thought about becoming a general surgeon. Any ideas about pursuing that particular option were beaten out of me during my days as a surgical dresser. Not by the workload, not by the patients, but by a consultant surgeon who met us every Wednesday at 8am to pass on pearls of wisdom.

After a couple of sessions about the anatomical relations of the spleen and the cutaneous nerve of the thigh, he felt he had drawn us into his thrall far enough to offer his views on the 'doctor–patient relationship'. In particular, the place of the digital rectal examination and its impact upon it.

He reminded us that the PR formed an essential part of any surgical examination. Quite how this opinion held water in, say, the ear, nose and throat clinic, was glossed over.

Not only did the rectal examination provide important diagnostic information, more importantly the vast majority of patients will do anything you tell them to do, take tablets twice a day without fail or stick to a diet of boiled fish – once you've had your finger up their bottom.

This profound insight into the complexity of the therapist–client dynamic was offered completely deadpan. I believe to this day that he meant every word. The best way to achieve high levels of treatment compliance from your patients was to make sure you'd got at least two knuckles somewhere near the recto-sigmoid junction at the first opportunity.

Later in life I discovered that this trick didn't only work on patients. Physiotherapists, staff nurses and hospital pharmacists all became incredibly co-operative and suggestible once their sphincters had been explored in those long, off-duty hours.

It's much more difficult to assess the beneficial effects of the anal probe in everyday general practice. I am currently in dispute with one of the establishments I visit regarding the re-writing of regular prescriptions. There's no computer system, and unlike my surgery, there are no reception staff to take on the mantle of slavishly copying last month's prescription list onto a new sheet.

Some of the nursing staff, when they have time, are willing to transcribe the repeats, otherwise it's down to my increasingly illegible scrawl and I live in fear of inadvertently changing Mrs Bloggs' daily metoprolol to metronidazole, or worse.

One of their number not only refuses to help out with the transcriptions, she refuses to dispense any medication not written in the doctor's own handwriting. Not just opiates – anything. She has been told by the Royal College of Nursing's legal team that if something went wrong with a prescription that she had issued, even though I had signed it, then she would be at risk because, unlike a receptionist, 'she ought to know what she's doing'. Even if nurses can't count, I thought they could at least copy in block capitals.

The vast majority of patients will do anything you tell them to – once you've had your finger up their bottom

But there it is: 'Catch 22B: Nurses cannot do anything they should know how to do. If they do it wrong, they might get into trouble.'

Time for the surgical probe again, and this time it's either proctoscope or rocket.

If patients can make it all up, so can I

I realise we're all supposed to be stressed out to the point of collective trichotillomania. But, if we're honest, isn't that feeling of tension often displaced by the even more uncomfortable sensation of boredom? Halfway through a standard afternoon surgery, I don't feel under pressure, I feel under-stimulated. You too? Then while away the tedium with a game I've invented.

This involves a slight extraction of urine from the punters, and I'm not talking Foley size 14s. My justification is that they started it. Every patient who's uttered the Large Person's Mantra, 'I don't eat a thing', has done it. So has anyone with a fractured fifth metacarpal caused by, 'Er . . . falling over'. And so has any asthmatic who swears compliance despite not having collected a prescription for 18 months.

Done what? Fabricated. Spouted bilge. Talked nonsense. This tendency to confabulate recently reached a bizarre peak when a woman presented with carpet burns to back and bottom. According to the patient, these were caused by a hedgehog that impaled itself when a friend had kicked it at her. While she was wearing a bikini. Yeah, right.

If patients can get away with talking cobblers for the sake of it, then, I reasoned, so can I. So I tried it out on the next lucky emergency surgery participant. Brett, aged seven, had hit his head on a wall. I know the child well: he's a yoblet from a family of boneheads. Frankly, it was the wall I felt sorry for.

'Was he,' I asked, 'knocked out?' No. 'Has he vomited?' No. 'Has he been drowsy?' No. I hesitated, unsure as to whether I could carry it off. 'Has he . . . has he started playing 'Bat Out Of Hell' by Meatloaf?'

'No,' the mother replied without missing a beat. And so I realised I could say what I liked to patients and get away with it – maybe because they assume I know what I'm doing, or because they're indulging me, or because they're simply not listening.

Admittedly, it may be that playing 'Bat Out Of Hell' by Meatloaf really is a sign of significant cranial trauma, and so might not have been such a dumb question after all. So I've tested my hypothesis by talking drivel on other occasions. And I can confirm it's risk-free, great fun and addictive.

Here's what I have asked in the last few days without provoking so much as a raised eyebrow. (1) Asked a patient with an in-growing toenail when she last had sex. *Answer*: Two days ago. (2) Asked someone with headaches, 'Is it like someone has ripped open your skull, torn your brain out and then pounded it into the ground with a sledgehammer?' *Answer*: A bit. (3) Asked a man with piles whether he wears his shirt tucked into his underpants. His reply was, 'No, would that help?' Well, I think it just might.

I realised I could say what I liked to patients and get away with it – maybe because they assume I know what I'm doing

Why a GP awareness week leaves me cold

Hang the flags out: it's National General Practice Week. You didn't know? Me neither. It's a sad irony that the organisers haven't managed to raise awareness in those they're trying to raise awareness of. So where do you suppose Dr Copperfield might stand on an event organised by the RCGP which hopes to 'promote and celebrate the strengths of family medicine and build stronger links with the public'? Just to one side, with boot raised. Because certain aspects do seem to deserve a good kicking.

For a start, National General Practice Week sounds alarmingly like one of those disease-awareness campaigns. And if there's one sure way to wind up a GP, it's with awareness weeks. We know they inevitably slap us round the face with the message: 'GPs should do more', conveniently overlooking the fact that generalists have to be vaguely 'aware' all the time rather than hyper-aware for just one week. So awareness campaigns make us shut our eyes and put our fingers in our ears.

But that's a posture which is hard to square with enthusiasm. And enthusiasm is what they're after. Otherwise, the college wouldn't brightly be suggesting, as part of the 'celebration', public debates, career talks for sixth-formers, sponsored bike rides and GPs working as receptionists, to name a few suggested jolly japes.

These ideas would be fine if we were a happy-clappy, fulfilled and motivated profession. But we're not. We're disenchanted, demotivated and depressed. In these circumstances, earnest enthusiasm falls flat: the balloon and badge brigade serve only to irritate and alienate. I'm not really going to put the boot in, though, because devoting a week to publicising general practice is actually a smart move. The college deserves a bouquet for having the idea, and for acting on it – but a brickbat for the content.

Look, if we really can grab the nation's attention for a week, let's make the most of it. Forget collaboration, let's be selfish for once, highlighting our problems of pay, status and workload.

Show our politicians how tough the job really is by getting them to shadow us for a day (and night). Drag pompous, sneering consultants from their ivory towers and give them shock treatment in the form of a surgery or two. Get a story in the papers highlighting how our preventive efforts save thousands of patients each year. Transmit some simple and effective health messages to the public using our media contacts – exploding myths about the 'urgency' of earache and the 'dangers' of simple fevers would reduce workload overnight.

If we really can grab the nation's attention for a week, let's be selfish for once and highlight our problems

'Too doctor-centred', the college and cardies will bleat. Precisely. Do something specifically for GPs for once, with no PC 'collaborative' or 'partnership' baggage – and patients will benefit. Why? Because GPs' morale will improve. And a happier GP is a safer, more functional GP.

But for us to grow in self-esteem, the college has to grow balls. And if they do, they'd better watch out – get it wrong next year, and I'll know exactly where to kick them.

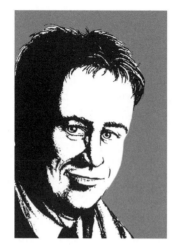

COPPERFIELD CALLING

. . . *the* *National* *Lottery*

Hello, National Lottery Press Office.

Hello, I wonder if you can help me. My name is Doctor Copperfield – I'm a GP in Essex. I'm just after some help regarding the National Lottery.

Of what sort?

Well, I understand that lottery winners are given all sorts of help and counselling to enable them to come to terms with a big win.

That's right, yes.

I just wondered if there was anything similar for persistent losers? You see, an awful lot of my patients go in for the lottery –

Really?

Yes, and they're getting progressively fed up about with not winning. They're all saying that . . . well . . . that it's a bit of a lottery really. But they're always moaning about it and I wondered if there was some type of help line for them?

Goodness me, I've never heard of this type of thing.

Oh yes, they're always going on about it. Is there no support group or something for them?

I'm not really sure.

I mean, some of them are spending so much on the lottery that they can't afford their prescriptions for antidepressants any more.

Oh dear. We don't really provide any help like that. From independent research, we find that the average spend per head is about two pounds, so people are playing in moderation, so we haven't really had a call for, you know . . . I've just never really heard of that before . . .

So if there's no support group, is there some other way to help? Could you arrange for some of them to have a small win, if I supplied you with names? Not the jackpot, just a tenner or something. To get them off my back.

Well, obviously, it's the luck of the draw, that's the whole point really, that's the idea of a lottery you know.

So what can I do with these sad losers then? What can I say to them? I've got a whole group of them and I promised I'd ring.

Well I don't know really . . . I mean a lot of my friends play quite regularly without any success, and then all of a sudden, you know, one sort of, I don't know, got four numbers or something the other week, so, you know, it can happen . . .

So keep trying?

Yes, I mean they've got a one in fifty four chance of winning any prize.

Well that's good, because I'm sure I've got at least fifty four of them, so on that basis one of them should win each week. I can tell them that, that might cheer them up a bit.

OK . . .

Anyway, have you got any tips for next week's numbers?

I haven't really . . . well . . . let's see . . . quite a few of the really big winners, how they've chosen their numbers is by making patterns on the ticket.

Really?

Yes, so tell them to try that. Making a pattern on their ticket.

Thanks for your help. Bye.

A heartsink by any other name . . .

One of the lesser known laws of physics, Copperfield's First Law of the Fat File, asserts that, no matter how fat a set of notes grows, the mass of the combined medical records, F, will never exceed the mass of the patient to whom they relate, K.

As F tends to infinity, so the corresponding variable, K, will increase in more or less direct proportion so that the ratio F/K will never equal or exceed unity.

In lay terms, most fat files detail the medical histories of obese patients. Invariably they are female and almost always over-investigated for trivial complaints, because nobody dares to sit down with them for a few minutes and explain that, for example, the human knee joint simply wasn't designed to sustain the weight of a fully grown rhinoceros. That's why the knee is (a) hurting like hell now and (b) will continue to hurt like hell for the foreseeable future, no matter how many X-rays and scans the orthopaedic surgeons can be bullied into ordering.

Some GPs call these patients 'heartsinks', others call them 'difficult to help'. I call them names and do my best not to harm them deliberately during the course of a consultation.

There really isn't any need to go out of my way to damage them proactively, as they will already be taking a combination of toxins prescribed by the barrage of consultants they've seen in outpatient clinics around the country. Many will be adding herbal or homoeopathic remedies into the mix, usually without telling any of their specialists for fear of causing offence, to ensure that the end result is either iatrogenic hepatotoxicity, cardiotoxicity or impaired renal function.

Now I am told by the shrinks that I have to stop labelling these people heartsinks or somatisers, even though these are well-recognised and extremely helpful parts of the medical lexicon. No, from now on these patients are to be told that they are suffering from chronic multiple functional somatic symptoms. Which means what, exactly?

Some of the time, and especially on the majority of occasions when I haven't a clue what the patient is on about, I simply translate the first three complaints or physical signs Mrs Lard mentions in the course of her twice-weekly dose of the doctor into fluent Medi-speak. Then I go on to explain that it's usually caused by a virus and to come back and see one of the trainees in a couple of weeks if things haven't improved.

I have been told by the shrinks to stop labelling patients heartsinks or somatisers – from now on, they are suffering from chronic multiple functional somatic symptoms

For example, when she tells me about those funny dizzy spells that start when she eats and are made worse by burping or passing urine, I hand over a bottle of pink gloopy medicine, tell her she's a textbook case of postprandial eructative labyrinthitis and show her the door. It never fails.

This is, of course, dishonest and total nonsense, but identical in essence to telling someone they have chronic multiple functional somatic symptom syndrome. Unlike Mrs Lard, who has a clear case of intractable poly-system psychogenic somatic complaint syndrome. Perhaps it's long-standing multi-focal non-organic somatic ailment syndrome. Or maybe it's everlasting pan-systemic supra-tentoria . . .

'snot like me to nurse a sniffle

All right, all right, I give up. No more jokes about nurses taking so many days off with minor illnesses that their regulatory body should be known as OFFSICK. No more articles about intrepid doctors injecting themselves with anti-nauseants before doing a full surgery plus walking wounded and visits when they ought to be throwing up salmonella-laden chicken korma in the privacy of their own bathroom.

You're all barmy.

No more gasps of awe either, when I hear tales of paramedics diving into pools of bodily fluids to site life-saving IV lines. No more pats on the back for physicians who wander through wards harbouring the Marburg bug, or any of the other bizarre viral haemorrhagic fevers people bring home with them from gap years in distant lands.

You're all mad.

There used to be a kind of unwritten law about all this. I go to work and meet hordes of snot-encrusted patients every week who haven't figured out that we don't have a cure for the common cold. Even if we had one, the NHS system of rationing (there, I said it) would ensure that only the privileged few would get their hands on prescriptions for the stuff, anyway.

They cough, splutter and throw up all over my chairs, carpets and clothes and in doing so expose me to a barrage of bacteria, viruses, protozoa and Christ knows what else in the course of my wonderful working day. Funnily enough, I don't remember catching anything serious from any of my patients. I got a nasty yeast infection from a physiotherapist once, but from my patients, nothing. So, I don't hate them any more when they're infectious than when they're not.

However, the *quid pro quo* has always been that if I did decide to roll up into work with a cold, the ailing masses would simply applaud my devotion to duty and take their chances, contagion-wise, without question.

Step forward Dr Helen Young, hospital doctor and caring kinda gal. Was she the type who would cancel a busy clinic because she had a sniffle? No way! She was right in there, diagnosing this, treating that, clerking routine surgical admissions and doing her best to mop up the green snot running from her nostrils with a pack of Kleenex clinical wipes. Dedication and plenty of it. Look and learn, nurses everywhere.

They cough, splutter and throw up all over my chairs, carpets and clothes and expose me to a barrage of bacteria and viruses

But – and this is a big but, a but so big it exerts a gravitational pull and has a small cluster of mini-buts orbiting around it – she didn't bank on meeting Trevor. Trevor was in for his pre-op assessment, and, horror of horrors, he caught her cold.

Now Trevor could have caught his cold on the bus on the way to hospital. He could have caught his cold from anyone in the waiting room, but he convinced our friends in the legal profession that he caught his cold from Dr Young. He sued Dr Young and was given £200 damages on a technicality after Dr Young and Salisbury District Hospital failed to respond to his complaint within 14 days.

So, well played Trevor and thank you. Because next time I so much as sneeze I'm off to my sickbed with the nurses. If you've got a case, they must have had it right all along.

My listening skills are tired and tested

I am a broken GP. For the first time ever, I've had to admit defeat in a consultation. Not bad after 14 years maybe, but a significant milestone on the road to Total Burnout.

First, some background. Mrs P is a somatiser. She's been merrily somatising all the time I've been here, and she somatised for my predecessor, too. Her frequently presented symptoms are many and varied, the only common thread being ever-present tiredness. Despite her ominous array of complaints, she remains well. Funnily enough, she's not a heartsink, as I know exactly where I stand with her. I've tried enlightening her about somatising (made her more tired), I know where I'm going with her (nowhere) and I know when to stop (as soon as possible). So, no problem. Until today.

'Doctor, you've got to do something about this tiredness.'

'Ah,' I say, flicking through the notes, 'You mean that tiredness which has been ever-present throughout your medical history?'

'That's the one,' she says, unabashed. 'I've had enough of it. My family says it's my hormones. And a friend reckons it could be my thyroid – and she's a first aider.'

I'm about to say that, being 15 years postmenopausal and a good 50 years post first episode of tiredness, hormones are unlikely to enter into the equation. And that it would be an awfully long time to have suffered an undetected thyroid problem, though, of course, who am I to argue with a sodding first aider – when she wades in with this:

'The thing is, doctor, I don't think you listen.'

Blimey! Insight! She's right. I don't listen and it's a good job, too. If I did, she'd have died of iatrogenesis years ago. Besides, it's not so much not listening as selectively not hearing the irrelevant white noise of her symptoms. Anything potentially serious my finely tuned antennae would pick up. Probably.

There ensues a very long consultation. After ten minutes, we've ironed out her misinterpretation of my tendency to nod off during her consultations. After 20, I've managed to explain to her the tightrope I walk: not over-investigating every symptom, as this might harm her, but not overlooking potentially serious problems either, as this might harm her, too.

By minute 25, she's even acknowledging that all this means I absorb some of her stress so that she suffers less, a fact I hadn't even realised myself. And by the half-hour mark, we're best buddies again.

Blimey! Insight! She's right. I don't listen and it's a good job, too. If I did, she'd have died of iatrogenesis years ago

'Thank you, doctor,' she says. 'I think I understand my symptoms much better now. There's just one last thing . . .' I look up. 'Can you do something about my dizziness? I've had it for years, so there must be something wrong . . .'

My world crumbles around me and I wave the white flag. 'What,' I ask, 'do you want me to do?' A thyroid test. Of course. By that point I'd have agreed to anything; I'd have eaten broken glass just to get her out of the room. I give her the form for the blood test. If those TFTs are abnormal, I resign.

The accompanying CD-ROM (originally distributed by *Doctor*) contains a selection of audio tracks from Tony Copperfield's column in *Doctor* and a screensaver that can be downloaded onto your PC. The audio tracks can be played through a standard CD player or through a PC if it is equipped with a sound card and speakers.

To listen to the tracks on a PC: insert the disk into CD-drive and click on Windows Start menu. Choose Programs>> Accessories>>Multimedia. Then choose CD-player.

To install the screensaver click on the Doctor Installer icon and the program will begin to install automatically. Windows Properties will control the screensaver. To open Properties, right click on your desktop and choose Properties>>Screensaver.

To uninstall the screen saver click on Windows Start menu. Choose Settings>>Control Panel>>Add/Remove programs. Select Doctor Screensaver, press add/remove button, and then press okay.

Licence Agreement
Licence Agreement Relating to *Tony Copperfield's Primary Care Scream* ('The Product') Published and distributed by Butterworth-Heinemann, an imprint of Elsevier Limited, and *Doctor* ('The Publisher') Attention! You are licensed to use the Product only upon the condition that you accept all of the terms in this Licence Agreement.

Licence
1. The Publisher grants you a non-exclusive, non-transferable personal licence on the terms of this Agreement to use and display the Product on a single computer on a single screen. The Product may not be installed on a network, or otherwise accessed or made accessible by more than one computer or computer screen.

Restrictions
2. You may not and you may not permit others to:
   (a) disassemble, decompile or otherwise derive source code from the Product or any part thereof
   (b) reverse engineer, reverse assemble, reverse compile or otherwise translate the Product or any part thereof
   (c) modify or prepare derivative works of or from the Product or any part thereof
   (d) copy the Product, except to make a single copy for archival purposes only
   (e) rent, lease, sell, distribute or sublicense the Product or any part thereof or make it available to any unauthorised persons
   (f) use the Product or any part thereof in any manner that infringes the intellectual property or other rights of another party
   (g) transfer the Product or any part thereof or any copy thereof to another party, unless you transfer all media and written materials in this package and retain no copies of the Software (including prior versions of the Software) for your own use
   (h) use the Product other than as specifically permitted in paragraph 1 above.

Term
3. This Licence is effective until terminated. You may terminate it at any time by destroying the Product, together with all copies and modifications of the whole or any part of the Product. This Licence may be terminated if you fail to comply with any term or condition of this Licence.

Limited warranty and limitation of liability
4. For a period of 60 days from the date that the Product is acquired by you, the Publisher warrants that the media upon which the Product resides will be free of defects that prevent you from loading the Product on your computer. The Publisher's sole obligation under this warranty is to replace any defective media, provided that you have given the Publisher notice of the defect within such 60-day period.

   The Publisher further warrants that your authorised use of or access to the Products pursuant to this Licence Agreement does not infringe any third party intellectual property rights.

   Except for such limited warranties, the Product is licensed to you on an 'AS IS' basis without any warranty of any nature. TO THE FULLEST EXTENT PERMITTED BY LAW, THE PUBLISHER DISCLAIMS ALL OTHER WARRANTIES, EXPRESS OR IMPLIED, INCLUDING WITHOUT LIMITATION THE IMPLIED WARRANTIES OF MERCHANTABILITY AND FITNESS FOR A PARTICULAR PURPOSE. THE PUBLISHER SHALL NOT BE LIABLE FOR ANY DAMAGE OR LOSS OF ANY KIND (INCLUDING WITHOUT LIMITATION INCIDENTAL, CONSE-QUENTIAL OR INDIRECT LOSS OR DAMAGE) ARISING OUT OF OR RESULTING FROM YOUR POSSESSION OR USE OF THE PRODUCTSOFTWARE (INCLUDING WITHOUT LIMITATION DATA LOSS OR CORRUPTION) OR ANY ERRORS OR OMISSIONS THEREIN, REGARDLESS OF WHETHER SUCH LIABILITY IS BASED IN TORT, CONTRACT OR OTHERWISE, WHETHER OR NOT FORESEEABLE, AND WHETHER OR NOT THERE IS AN ADEQUATE ALTERNATIVE REMEDY. FURTHERMORE, TO THE FULLEST EXTENT PERMITTED BY LAW, ALL RESPONSIBILITY IS SPECIFICALLY DISCLAIMED BY THE PUBLISHER FOR ANY INJURY AND/OR DAMAGE TO PERSONS OR PROPERTY AS A RESULT OF THE USE OR OPERATION OF ANY IDEAS, INSTRUCTIONS, PROCEDURES OR METHODS CONTAINED IN THE PRODUCTS. YOUR SOLE REMEDY IS THE REFUND OF ANY FEES PAID FOR ACCESS TO THE PRODUCT. IF THE FOREGOING LIMITATION IS HELD TO BE UNENFORCE-ABLE, THE PUBLISHER'S MAXIMUM LIABILITY TO YOU SHALL NOT EXCEED THE AMOUNT OF THE LICENCE FEES PAID BY YOU FOR THE SOFTWARE. THE REMEDIES AVAILABLE TO YOU AGAINST THE PUBLISHER UNDER THIS AGREEMENT ARE EXCLUSIVE. SOME STATES DO NOT ALLOW THE LIMITATION OR EXCLUSION OF IMPLIED WARRANTIES OR LIABILITY FOR INCIDENTAL OR CONSEQUENTIAL DAMAGES, SO THE ABOVE LIMITATIONS OR EXCLUSIONS MAY NOT APPLY TO YOU.

   If the information provided in the Product contains medical or health sciences information, it is intended for professional use within the medical field. Information about medical treatment or drug dosages is intended strictly for professional use, and because of rapid advances in the medical sciences, independent verification of diagnosis and drug dosages should be made.

Publisher's rights
5. United Kingdom and international copyright and all other proprietary rights in the Product and materials supplied to you as part of this package belong to the Publisher. You expressly agree that the Product contains information con-fidential to the Publisher. You agree to take all reasonable steps to protect the Publisher's copyright and confidential information notice, including without limitation retaining the appropriate notices on anyll copyies or modifications of the Product made for archival purposes. You will also agree that you will not recompile the object code provided to you, or use any other technique to produce a source-code version of this Product.

General
6. You may not sublicense, transfer or assign this Licence.
7. This Licence will be governed by English law.
8. You acknowledge that you have read and understand this Licence and agree to be bound by its terms and conditions. You further agree that it is the complete and exclusive statement of the agreement between us which supersedes any proposal or prior agreement, oral or written, between us relating to the subject matter of this Licence.
9. Failure to comply with any provision shall be grounds for termination of this Licence.

Copyright Notice
10. Copyright of *Tony Copperfield's Primary Care Scream* rests with the Publisher. You may not distribute copies. The reproduction of the entire Product or substantial extracts from such requires the separate written permission of the Publisher.